HEAVY LIGHT

Non-fiction

Running for the Hills

Truant: Notes from the Slippery Slope

Sicily: Through Writers' Eyes

A Single Swallow

Down to the Sea in Ships

Orison for a Curlew

Myths and Legends of the Brecon Beacons

Icebreaker

The Light in the Dark: A Winter Journal

Something of his Art: Walking to Lübeck with J. S. Bach

Fiction

The Prince's Pen

For Children

Aubrey and the Terrible Yoot

Aubrey and the Terrible Ladybirds

Heavy Light

A Journey Through Madness, Mania and Healing

HORATIO CLARE

Chatto & Windus
LONDON

3 5 7 9 10 8 6 4 2

Chatto & Windus, an imprint of Vintage

Chatto & Windus is part of the Penguin Random House
group of companies whose addresses can be found at
global.penguinrandomhouse.com

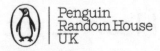

Penguin
Random House
UK

First published by Chatto & Windus in 2021

penguin.co.uk/vintage

Quotes on pp. 235 & 236 from Rehling, J. & Moncrieff, J. (2020), 'The
functions of an asylum: an analysis of male and female admissions to the
Essex County Asylum in 1904', *Psychological Medicine*, 15 January, 2020.

Quotes on pp. 272 & 273 from Arkowitz, H. & Lilienfeld S. O. (2012),
'EMDR: Taking a Closer Look', *Scientific American
Special Editions* 17, 4s, 10–11, August 2012.

Quote on p. 318 from Deegan, P. E. (2004), 'Remember My Name:
Reflections on Spirituality in Individual and Collective Recovery', keynote
address at the University of Kansas, Lawrence Kansas, p. 4.

A CIP catalogue record for this book is available from
the British Library

ISBN 9781784743529

Typeset in 11.5/13.75 pt Ehrhardt MT
by Integra Software Services Pvt. Ltd, Pondicherry

Printed and bound in Great Britain by Clays Ltd, Elcograf S.p.A.

The authorised representative in the EEA is Penguin Random House
Ireland, Morrison Chambers, 32 Nassau Street, Dublin D02 YH68.

Penguin Random House is committed to a sustainable future for
our business, our readers and our planet. This book is made from
Forest Stewardship Council® certified paper.

MIX
Paper from
responsible sources
FSC
www.fsc.org   FSC® C018179

For Rebecca – because there are no words.

If I should fall from grace with God
Where no doctor can relieve me . . .

Shane MacGowan

Contents

Author's note

Sometimes my memory flashes up a scene, an exchange, something I said or did, and I flinch in horror and shame. *But how* on earth *could you possibly have believed* any *of it?* I think. Yet it was not a question of belief. It was what was. The whole thing was as real as a full stop on a page.

This is the story of how I went mad, how I was treated, how I got better and of what I know, now, about how we deal with madness and breakdown. A personal journey through society, psychiatry and psychotherapy, this book seeks understanding of a widespread crisis, which shame and fear have tended to conceal.

There are different terms for what I experienced. The plainest is madness, which descends through Old English from the Latin, *mutare*, 'to change', and the proto-Germanic *gamaidaz*, 'changed for the worse'.

As we shall see, the diagnosis, treatment and monetisation of all the different forms of 'changed for the worse' that we now experience has made the language of these conditions slippery and treacherous.

According to a model which treats madness as you would a disease, we begin the story in mania and travel through psychosis to recovery (there is no cure). Another perspective has it that this is a story of extreme distress which moves through crisis into healing (there is no end).

They agree on psychosis – a technical term in the disease model for a state involving hallucinations and delusions. Another way of understanding psychosis is to take its Greek meaning, 'sick of soul', literally. I would ask my reader to hold both these perspectives in mind as you witness behaviour which might otherwise seem inexplicable, or all too explicable.

This aims to be a straightforward story. I hope it might offer some help, hope and insight to those who suffer breakdowns and to those who love and care for them.

PART I

CHAPTER 1

Signs and wonders

Manchester airport in December, rain spittles the early-morning dark. In Terminal 3 lines of families with baggage trolleys queue up in matched sets. I skim around check-in fetching coffee for my partner, croissants and fruit for the boys. I smoke outside, feeling like a pirate impostor in what looks to me like a bourgeois festival of skiing, of happy families and decorum. With clumsy sleight of hand I conceal a knuckle of hash in my hold bag.

My partner, Rebecca, and her elder son, Robin, seventeen, are wary of me. They look suspicious and irritated. I am ebullient. I dismiss the worry and reproof in their faces. I am on holiday at last. Aren't we all on holiday? Haven't I earned a bit of folly? Over the last months I have published and publicised two new books, started a new job and crossed and recrossed the country speaking in bookshops and festivals.

Steadily, as autumn turned to winter, I have risen through feelings of optimism and energy into hypomania. Hypomania describes an excited state of elevated mood. It is characterised by flights of ideas, surges of vitality, sleeplessness and irritability. In this state it feels natural to spend incautiously, to begin new relationships and make exciting plans. Mildly alarming to friends and family, hypomania brings with it dash, wit and charisma. People can be drawn to its light and glamour. I had taught well, putting immense effort and belief

into my students. At my book events I had evangelised for
an understanding of cyclothymia (a mild form of bipolar,
from which I suffer) and seasonal affective disorder; I felt
charged with a significant mission, even as my condition
intensified. The light by which I felt surrounded, the light
I threw and reflected, became an alarming glare.

Hay, Cambridge, Manchester, Chester, Halifax, Cardiff,
London, Felixstowe, Bath, London again and back and forth
to Hebden and Manchester . . . I have done longer tours,
but this was a yo-yo of constant journeys out and back. I
split the soles of my feet until they bled, lost my voice and
contributed to many magazines, newspapers and radio
programmes while clinging to a resolution to make it home
to Yorkshire at the end of each night.

My diary from this period is an eloquent record of a crazed
attempt to be everywhere at once. Not recorded there are
my internal staccatos – perfectionism, ambition, inadequacy,
guilt – or my secret strategy. I was using cannabis as a
stimulant and, with drink, a tranquilliser.

I know cannabis has a history of making me manic but I
have been happy to pay that price in return for the energy
hypomania grants. I will stay on top of it all, of course. I am
done, now, finished with this huge effort of work. I can lay
off and relax. Everything will be fine. This holiday is
Rebecca's idea. She has arranged and paid for it.

She knows how hard I have been working. She has watched
me becoming hypomanic since November, seen my optimism, my energy and my sleeplessness accumulating. She is
thinking that if she can just get us all to the mountains we
will be able to relax. She is hoping that being outside in the
snow and air, away from work and pressure, will help me to
calm down.

In the queues I horse around with our son, five, who is
also excited. He gauges the tension between Daddy and
Mummy. They argue sometimes but they love each other,

he knows, and everyone loves him. He is especially happy because his brother, whom he worships, is with us. At security Rebecca and the children go through while my backpack is turned aside for searching. I wait in the security zone, perching up on the repacking table, surveying the queues, the cameras, the searchers, the scanners, the conveyors, the trays and the passengers, and I begin to play the game. I know it *is* a game, on one level, but as soon as I begin to play it becomes real.

Notice that man touching his hat, indicating that person over there making a strange flicking gesture? Follow the gesture and you come to that young woman's raised hand – she's pretending to stretch but now she looks far across the room at that chap, who catches the flick and passes it to the sharp-looking woman over there who nods it to the military-looking man over here, who returns it to me, and with a thump of my heart and a twitch I quickly pass it on, glancing it to the man there who tics it over to the security supervisor who nods and shrugs it on to the woman beside him who glances across the room – and round we go again. And it ends with the woman in the NASA T-shirt, who seems to confirm it all with a look straight at me.

NASA – you could not ask for a more definite sign! Some game is afoot and I am definitely part of it. Just imagine, *imagine* being part of some great and secret scheme; imagine being trained to observe, to communicate and relay signals by means covert but unmistakable. I can't wait to find out more, to play on, to do my part.

If you had taken me out of the room and sat me down and asked me what I was thinking, and if I had answered honestly, I would have said that I thought there really could be something exciting and concealed taking place.

I would have suggested that the tour company that Rebecca had selected may partly be a front for some kind of government agency. Some or many of us on the plane may be among an elect, including former soldiers and employees of the shadow state. And if they are, then I am especially marked out. I am being carefully watched. As a journalist-observer-participant, I may have a crucial role to play in what is to come.

This is not the first time this winter that I have harboured secret fantasies and forgotten they were fantasies. There have been encounters: I really have had strange and possibly not coincidental contact with a communicator for the Chinese government. I really did meet influential Moroccan dissidents on a recent assignment to Italy. These meetings give my dream-game real characters and rooted stories. I am craving signs of more. The interludes in which I can stop playing are becoming very short.

My bag passes the check. Rebecca spotted the not-so-sleight of hand and has been thinking I must have been arrested. Rather than acknowledge her anger and alarm I brush her off.

I cannot ski and do not feel any great attraction to ski culture but I am looking forward to it on my family's behalf. And I am looking forward to the food, to the coffee, to the mountains, to Italian, to a thriller in an Alpine setting, to a world turning, to characters I love, to the walk-ons and cameos. I sense conspiracy waiting like a gun under a coat. Reality and fantasy turn somersaults inside me. I believe I can pass as normal but there is a jangle about me. People sense it. The eyes of other passengers on the plane linger for giveaway, assessing moments. We are almost subliminally sensitive to the currents of others' minds, to something, to anything not quite right.

On the approach to Innsbruck I wake and look out on a mountain of a height and scale I have never seen. As my son and I stare out I feel a kind of vertigo, a thudding thrill. This is an unearthly mountain, something from a sci-fi film, too high and huge to be real, but right there, unarguable. We tilt and the view realigns. The aircraft is banking, that is all. What appeared vertical is horizontal. But I am seized by the glimpse of the world on a skewed plane, which made it extraordinary, previously unseen. Now as we switch and turn through the valleys we are being shown the terrain, given a preview of the theatre of operations.

CHAPTER 2

Mania

O ut into the lucent air at Innsbruck we go. I snatch a very small joint in the car park – fragments of crumbs of cannabis – and cannot tell if it makes any difference to the splendid definition of the peaks, to the blue bright sky and the joy of being abroad. We are driven over the Italian border and up into the Dolomites. The rep from our tour company, Joe, is a kind and steady man, a Yorkshireman, as it happens. He and the driver confer.

'Can we take the pass? Have they opened it?'

Opened it for us? I think.

'Yes!'

They rejoice. We are privileged somehow. Someone is looking out for us, opening roads for us. We zigzag up the pass to the top where the snow is luxurious, lying in deep sparkling blankets on either side.

'Look! Look at the snow, darling! Isn't it wonderful! Isn't it magical?

'Yes, Dad!'

'And look at *that* . . .'

A peak like a shard of fallen planet towers above us. Our driver, Alex, is a local, a Ladin, intense behind the wheel. He steers us through hairpins which twist down to a valley where villages glow, lamplit in the dusk and frigid air. The descent into the valley is a masterclass in control, the vehicle snarling in low gear, slaloming down through the pine forest, Alex's concentration absolute, my little boy beside me, both of us thrilled. At nightfall we arrive at the Hotel Medil, a hefty chalet at the foot of the mountains in the village of Campitello di Fassa.

In the story I tell myself afterwards there were sane interludes in the Medil. We manage the dinner on the first night together. We swim in the pool and use the spa without incident. There are quiet times in the bar. Our fellow guests include Simon, a tall tanned Brit with the voice and bearing of an officer. He is something in the special forces, I decide, on 'our' team. Simon is travelling with his son and daughter. His son is surely something to do with GCHQ – he is keeping tabs on everything through his phone – and his daughter must be on her way to joining a plain-clothes army intelligence unit. I get drunk with Simon. In the morning I give him back his wallet and the plug from his bathroom basin. I am not clear how I came by them.

We have booked a family room. I am obnoxious and irrational. Wearing socks and trying to move the bunk bed I kick it; the nail of my right big toe is torn to the root. Rebecca insists I take my own room. In here I spend the nights drinking, smoking, talking to the mirror, to the TV, obsessing over the Internet and the news, barely sleeping.

But Rebecca remembers this:

'On the second night they brought you up from the bar. They said, "He's obviously really drunk." I went down to speak with them. You'd really hurt your toe – the nail was hanging off, and Robin was bandaging it. You were crying, you were really distraught, and you gave him a diatribe about me. You were really explicit, just the most horrible things. And he was hugging you and saying it's all right Horace, you just need to go to sleep. But when I came back up you locked yourself in the bathroom and started dragging things off the shelves and throwing things around. So then I had to say to the hotel guys actually, I do need help, I need another room. They said do you want us to call the police? Robin went down and spoke to them – he said, don't do that, this is mental health, and he tried to explain to them in Italian what the problem was. He got them to look it up and he rang Giovanni [a friend, a psychiatrist in Verona], who explained it to them too. And the hotel guys were so lovely. They took pity on me and the boys. They said your family are lovely, the hotel's quiet, you can have the other room for free . . .'

I wake knowing there was a row last night and that I caused it but I am more defiant than embarrassed. There is something much more important going on. News comes from Britain that mysterious sightings of drones have closed Gatwick Airport. I do not believe they are drones (in fact the details of the incident remain somewhat obscure). The airport is being buzzed by craft belonging to a superior technology. The drone story is a cover-up; events are moving very quickly. Humanity is being asked to prove that we can unite and work together. I have no doubt that some of the world's governments have been contacted by a superior civilisation, threatened – at Gatwick and probably elsewhere – and challenged to come up with a unified response.

What is happening in the Ladin Alps, in the Val di Fassa, takes on extreme importance. Here representatives of different nations engage in war games and winter sports, demonstrating understanding between nations through cooperation. Everyone is going all-in – there can be no holding back: the planet and our children's futures are at stake, so demonstrating family cohesion is important too. My parenting involves bringing tea and fruit to the family's room, feeling aggrieved that this does not cut any ice with Rebecca or Robin, playing with our son in the pool, playing in the snow, riding the odd ski bus with him, applauding from a distance as he masters skiing, and otherwise keeping – and being kept – well clear.

In my room I follow the story on television, every programme slithering with subtext and messages for me. Studying the number plates of tourists' cars, I realise that the many vehicles with Czech plates have been hired by Russians. The young couple who say they are from Ukraine, Yuri and Ivana, must be in charge of the Russian side, possibly delegates from the Kremlin. Simon is all but confessing to being a senior officer in the Special Air Service. Neither he nor the Ukrainian couple want to sit near us – near me – at dinner any more, but we meet outside to smoke.

'Don't you think there's something odd about Joe?' Simon says of our tour company rep, the gentle and stalwart Yorkshireman, who has not been to this valley before.

'Royal Marines Mountain Troop,' I say with complete conviction.

Simon says nothing and turns away, swallowing. It is quite possible that some manic perceptions are accurate, of course. I would still bet that Simon had been in the army at some point, even if he was no longer.

The barman is a member of the Italian intelligence services. The receptionist from Moldova is a Russian. The hotel next door, where many Russians are staying, is the base of our competitors, whom we must make our friends. The retired teacher from Liverpool who was on our plane is a senior member of British intelligence. I must demonstrate solidarity with all sides, all the time.

In the heights around us, unseen between the black pine trees, on the near-vertical screes among the glowing snow and murderous rock, elite soldiers move unseen, training their cross hairs on us and each other, war gaming, overseeing, awaiting orders, protecting and menacing. Their leaders in NATO and the Kremlin have sensibly agreed to replace actual conflict with secret tournaments. My role is exhausting but I am full of vim for it.

In the mornings I first aim to see the family off without getting into a fight with Rebecca or Robin. Then I must move between the bars for coffee, cigarettes and quite soon drinks, being equally respectful of the powers each represents. Nothing and nowhere is only itself: every establishment belongs to a tribe, to a competing set of interests I must win over or appease. For example, in the Albergo Agnello, Ladin farmers in conical hats drink coffee and shots of spirits. Here too are the kinds of old men I know from Sicily, old men with eyes locked in faces of iron blankness, old men with secrets. You deal with the Mafia — for there can surely be no peace on earth without the cooperation of organised crime — by showing perfect manners to the hostess, by evincing a humble manner and bearing, by leaving a tip which is neither too large nor too small, by counting the merest nod in response to your greeting as a concession, and by remaining impassive when you are snubbed.

Now on to the Bar Evita, the centre of women's power in the village, where I might order half a Guinness and submit to inspection and cordial mockery by the black-eyed rumbustious lady in charge. Here good grace, good humour and humility are called for. Straight white men know where they stand in the resolution of the battle of the sexes: very quietly, very humbly, lucky to be alive. In the Evita it is important to be most respectful, and to get the tip exactly right.

The Evita is also a meeting place. On the day the news breaks that Donald Trump has dismissed General Jim Mattis as secretary of defense, a heavy American with an aura of powerful self-possession strides in. I do not know if he is here to look me over — he does — or if I should evaluate him. I do. We nod and hold each other's gaze. Some assessment has taken place at some senior level. Some agreement has

been reached. An element in the American defence establishment wishes me to know that I am known.

I spend much time checking different euro coins – the
nationalities of the coins are part of another subsystem.
Proudly Tyrolese native German speakers might prefer
German coins, as Italians might their own, and when in doubt
there are always the neutral Dutch, French or Greek coins.

Obsessive ritual is a feature of this stage of my mania. It
is addictive and absorbing. I accumulate different versions
of patterns I have to fulfil until my every moment is beset
by rituals to enact, by different calls on my time and attention, as though I am playing multiple games of chess at once.
So, cigarette stubs in an ashtray must be left in a star pattern.
Certain drinks must be balanced with others. In order to
maintain harmony, I must perform the same sequences in
different places. I must assure and placate every barman,
waiter, customer and tourist. To be constantly doing, to be
ever in action, makes a fine defence against any other inter-
pretation of the way I am behaving.

Up the road in Canazei is a bar frequented by ski instruc-
tors, climbers and sportspeople. I am sure that the woman
behind the bar, Paola, is a veteran of an Italian parachute unit,
injured in battle. The men are military aged, fit, often encum-
bered with sophisticated gear. Here I eat, drink, tip, write,
leave patterns of cigarettes, clear glasses from the outside
tables, practise the runic tribute system of the coins and settle
in, finding it impossible to stay at any table for long.

Above us the mountains are living giants and slumbering
dragons, pulsing theatres of snow and light. Along the ridges
tiny sticks are ski lifts. In the evening white fountains jump
along these skylines. Smoke bombs set off by triumphant
commandos or snowblowers gilding the runs? Both.
Sometimes I have to be brave. Sometimes the sniper's bullet
is only a finger-squeeze away. Mostly I just have to be calm,
to ride my surging tides, to pass as normal. I find a place of

safety in the Bar Regina, under the large and sympathetic eyes of a tender man whose assertively camp manner and kohled eyes suggested a confident position outside the valley's norms. We talk about little things – the valley, the tourist seasons, who I am and what I am doing, nothing much. Italians draw understanding and security from seeing people in the company of family or friends. A lone, eagerly gregarious figure in a resort village might not be a wolf but is not quite a benign presence either. My odder behaviour I try to keep out of sight.

Visiting the village church, I fall into desperate sobbing over the small graves of children. Testing my nerve and judgement, I follow covert assault courses, inching and jumping across fantastic varieties of ice, firn and frozen snow. My version of skiing is a lot of fun, it turns out.

The hotel is an exciting place. There is a toy moose on a table in the hall with cameras for eyes. Motion sensors on the stairs conceal cameras. Mirrors and TV screens observe you.

In the crowded and observant dining room the buffet is a test. Each of the many platters represents the claims of a different clan, culture or country. I cannot be seen to favour any, so concoct strange hybrids under the alarmed eyes of the maître d'.

'Salad in your soup?' Rebecca cries. 'Really?'

I cannot explain, of course. A pugnacious defiance becomes my mode of dealing with her. 'It's delicious. You should try it.'

I am a despicable shit.

Her despairing concern I take for hostility and resentment – and partly, since my behaviour is wrecking a holiday with our children that she has worked very hard and saved for – it is. There is a crisis over the passports: where have I hidden them? There is another over socks – why have I taken Robin's? There are my postings on social media. One, meant only partly in jest, says I hate skiing and am out of money: could

anyone who owes me any please pay up? Those who see it react
with alarm, amusement or incredulity. My father is horrified.
What on earth do I think I am doing, writing something like
that in an 'obscenely public' space?

I have no idea how hard Rebecca is working to keep the
holiday afloat, me out of jail and the hotel calm. It says a lot
about Rebecca that she manages to laugh as she recalls it.

'So every night when you came into the restaurant one of
the waiters and the maître d' would come over and say,
"Would you like salad in your soup, Mr Horatio?" They
were just absolutely wonderful. And they'd just stand by our
table when you were there, though you never stayed very long.

'And there was a Ukrainian couple and you kept speaking
Russian to them – and they asked you not to speak it, they
were really offended by it. But we explained. And that lovely
English family, they moved away and made it clear they
weren't moving away from us – but from you . . .'

Madness of this kind is like a sunrise of the self, a flood
of light banishing the shadows of the relative, of perspective.
My sun is rising fast, strobing the world with new colours
until it glows in hyperreality. I feel myself infused with this
light, which feels like knowledge and power and significance;
a light which seems tangible and almost visible to others,
judging by the way they look at me. It is like being famous,
not in the slight ways writers might be famous, but
Hollywood-film-star famous. It is exhilarating and exhausting,
but the exhaustion, the weight of this spotlight, I push away
constantly, in the same way I brush away the miserable
tension in my family as a series of normal arguments, as
Rebecca and Robin ganging up on me, as a bit too much to
drink, as nothing much.

One evening we get through supper, I say goodnight to
the children and Rebecca and return to the bar. There are
few other residents present, mercifully. I begin to drink beer
and whisky. The dapper young Nicolo is on duty. He is

bright and charismatic; immaculately dressed in his blazer, he looks like a male model. His service is delivered with flourishes of sardonic humour. Nicolo is not destined to be a barman but he is impersonating one with elan. It is unfortunate that one of his customers partly believes him to be a member of the Italian domestic intelligence service, inadequately hiding his real profession and purpose.

I like him immediately. Normally I would be able to recount something of his background, his education, his plans and hopes, but I do not ask Nicolo the questions I normally ask, being too busy with myself and my world-saving. We toss coins and compete for the highest number on a mini roulette wheel. I offer him drinks. He serves mine. At some point we begin to talk about rugby. In my mind rugby is also a metaphor for the different competing teams on the mountains and in the hotels around us, for the governments dealing and jostling in the background, for the great secret endeavour to unite the world. We are all joined in a great global challenge; the future of humanity is at stake, a better, fairer, united world the prize.

'We can do it! We must do it! We can win! And if you try to stop us we will smash you, mate!'

Suddenly I am standing on the bar's footrail, looming up over Nicolo, red in the face and shouting in Italian. I have no idea how it happened. I have never behaved this way before. Nicolo is frightened and amazed. I am spitting water at him.

All at once Davide is there, huge, bull-like Davide, a saturnine man who works on reception at night, his shoulders and arms swelling his smart shirt. Davide seizes me and rushes me out of the bar. I offer no resistance. I am limp with confusion – what is going on? Davide drags me across the lobby floor into the space between the inner and outer doors. He holds me over the doormat, gripping the throat of my shirt, his heavy fist bunched and hovering over my nose.

'Call the Carabinieri,' I say evenly, and again, 'Call the Carabinieri.'

'Listen, *cazzo*. This is my valley, this is my village, there's no Carabinieri, there's no police, there's nothing in the world that will protect you from me and my friends,' Davide retorts. I think the level of his fury surprises us both. I apologise. I feel utter bewilderment. I am calm. After an emphatic shake Davide releases me. I apologise again and I go to my room. What was that about?

By morning I can explain the whole thing. I was spiked. At the instruction of the unseen powers directing the operation, the last drink Nicolo served me concealed a powerful chemical designed to blast my levels of adrenaline, testosterone and aggression off the charts. It was like stepping into an elevator and finding yourself in a rocket. The point was to discover how I would react to the sudden threat of physical violence. By remaining calm and rational, by asking for the Carabineri, by mollifying Davide, by not panicking, I have passed with distinction.

'I was spiked,' I reassure Rebecca. 'It was a test. I passed. They didn't mean any harm. He even held me over the mat, so it was soft – the whole thing was fake.'

Rebecca looks appalled. There are no words that can help us. All she can do is keep the children away from me and try to contain my flailing.

I apologise to Nicolo and Davide. We are elaborately courteous and cordial for the rest of the week. I feel great affection for both of them, honestly believing they were doing as instructed. 'They feel very bad about it,' I tell Rebecca, 'but it's completely fine. They were only doing what they were told. We're friends.'

To two proofs – UFOs over Gatwick, and this operation, this sneaky but no doubt necessary test of nerve – add a third. With mordant timing, the conspiracy now sends a friend from Verona, Kay, to the hotel. (Or rather, Kay and

Rebecca arrange that she will come up and see us, as we are
all beloved friends.) Like many US expats in the Veneto,
Kay *is* in fact connected to an arm of the American defence
establishment. Kay's husband was in the US military for
many years. Not party to classified intelligence but inevitably
a witness to some of her husband's doings, Kay is entirely
discreet about their adventures. It was a standing joke that
when her husband visited her in Verona she would not see
us; we never met him. Her presence now is proof of all that
I suspect and believe. My role is to show friendship and
solidarity with the United States – she will surely be reporting
back on us and me – and to make sure she comes to no harm.

My room is a relentless theatre. On my balcony I can be
watched or shot by dozens of unseen observers. The Russians
in the adjoining hotel, whose windows and balconies face
mine, are monitoring me. Television programmes contain
messages for me; the Internet is a swamp of surveillance,
covert messaging and exposure.

Following the news on English, French and Italian channels, I try to stay on top of it all. I deliver long monologues
to the bathroom mirror: 'We can do it!' I roar. 'We can come
together, we can! We can change. We can *do this*! I know we
can, I believe in us . . .'

Above all I am concerned about the drones at Gatwick. If
we do not make progress with our secret cooperations and
competitions, our negotiations and dealings, we will invite a
much more destructive demonstration of extraterrestrial
power. Something terrible is coming, I can feel it. All this
is ending, will end, if we do not change our ways
dramatically.

I realise what I must do. I must be brave. Every time I
stand on the balcony I know I can be picked off, but I open
the curtains and the windows and angle my laptop at the
stars. At top volume I begin to broadcast the signal that the
Sputnik sent to earth. Its staccato bleeps and static reassure

the overseeing spacecraft that things are going well, that we
are making progress.

First contact has been made, and recently, I would guess.
The governments of the earth are under mighty pressure to
reach agreements. Perhaps the Sputnik signal will buy us a
little more time. I am thoroughly and luridly sick on the
balcony, expelling volumes of wine-red vomit. I soak it up
with towels which I leave outside. Overnight they freeze into
rigid pink sheets. Somehow this seems to offset the malignant
symbolic power of the Coca-Cola cans on my balcony.

In the morning the Dolomites rupture up, steaming with
frost wisps. The pines are black against the sky. Sunrays are
blades of exhilarated light, slicing blue shadows. Out into it,
muffled and crunching the snow, vivid with the intensity of
the day, I walk with Kay.

We have known each other a long time. Kay drove us to
hospital the night Rebecca's waters broke. We have a kind
friendship, yet this morning we are wary of each other, as if
we carry weapons in holsters. As well as being a lovely, funny,
loyal friend, Kay is the self-possessed, military-backed might
and certainty of the United States, suspicious of me but, so
far, benign.

'Shall we go there?' she says.

'Sure.'

'I'm so worried about you, Horatio. Are you OK?'

'Of course I am, dear Kay!'

My main concern is to protect her. She must be very on
edge, after the briefings she has had. Being in the middle of
this nest of soldiers and spies and journalists at a critical time
for humanity . . . and being given a specific task and people
to answer to, rather than the free-ranging role I have: I would
not fancy it. I wish I could unburden myself to her but of
course it is out of the question.

I walk with K as her bodyguard, assessing every window,
face and passing car for threat. I want to show all the rival

powers that the military of Trump's America can be reasonable, can be considered vulnerable and treated as friendly.
We sit together. I ask about her family.

I look on Kay with deep affection and scepticism. No
doubt the US is trying for some advantage by sending her
into this crucible with me. I must be unwavering in my
refusal to be drawn out, in my determination to show no
special favour. But at the same time I love Kay and what she
stands for, which is pride in her family and her friends, and
generosity and humour and iconoclasm in all the best
American ways. Whatever else they say about the Special
Relationship, we do get each other's jokes.

'Oh, Horatio, I'm so worried about you. Are you OK? I
don't think you are really . . .'

'I'm fine. Really I am – I'm fine!'

'Rebecca's so worried about you.'

'I know. I'm very sorry about it but there is nothing I can
do. My therapist says I take on too much responsibility for
other people's feelings.'

'But you are responsible for her feelings! A bit – a *lot* –
aren't you?'

'I know. She takes on so much – everything. I wish she
would go for counselling but she won't.'

'But this is isn't about her, is it? What about you?'

'I'm fine! How is it going with you?'

'I'm fine too!' she laughs.

'Really? Everything is all right?'

'Well *yes*, I think so . . .'

She looks tender and grave. So really, then, the Americans
are all in, too. They have their worries, I can see them on
her face, but really, *it is all fine*. So far.

I feel such relief. I feel tremendous.

Kay has to leave and I must make redress, must balance
this contact with her. Next door is the hotel which is serving
as the Russian headquarters; many of the cars parked outside

have Czech plates. I visit their spa. In the gym is a Russian trainer; we exchange friendly greetings. Downstairs are hard-bodied men and women exercising, steaming and swimming with their children. I join them. Some of the children in the pool are Russian and I greet them in their language. They and their parents are easy and cordial with me. I use the gym, the sauna, the pool. I let them see that I am unafraid and not to be feared. So far, things are going well. All is in harmony.

Simon the soldier is stressed, worried about his flight back to Gatwick. I offer him accommodation with us: 'If you're stuck, fly to Manchester, you can stay with us for as long as you like.' He is cordial. Then we fall to discussing Brexit. For the first time he comes close to losing his temper. We are on different sides of this argument.

'I think the EU is one of humanity's great achievements,' I say. 'I think we should extend its borders to Cape Town and Novosibirsk. What we want is a global EU.'

'I don't fucking believe it!' he shouts. 'That's so ridiculous. How can you possibly believe that?'

His vehemence confirms my belief that what I think matters and will have consequences with our superiors.

Tangled through the roots of mania and psychosis is this recurring dream of significance. It is as though I am newly born in the world, craving meaning and interaction as I once craved milk and contact. I will do nearly anything to satisfy that need, from terrorising myself to ranting in the street.

More guests arrive at the hotel. I do my porter/bodyguard bit, helping them in with their things. Every night I do security rounds of the hotel, making sure the perimeter is safe. I check the basements and storage areas for bombs and points of vulnerability. Ironically, having a lunatic staying with them probably renders the Medil's guests as safe as they have ever been.

Running like a tide against a great and rather terrible need to be known for who I think I really am is an awareness that there is something wrong with me in the eyes of others, which leads me to conceal what I really think.

Underlying my relief at the appearance of Kay, and the comfort I take from powers watching me and shadowy people knowing about me, is the knowledge that I am valued. How wonderful to have no secrets. How wonderful, in a way, to be vetted and studied by the security services, to be known fully, better than my family and best friends know me, better than I know myself – the ultimate cure for existential isolation.

In the mental hospital where I will end up, some of my most lucid fellow patients will tell me about themselves, reveal and unload their histories, their achievements, the stories of what they had done and become, scrabbling to reassert the worth of their lives to a world which judges us fit only – as we see it when we are inside – to be locked away. In the absence of any talking therapy in the hospital, we did what we could to improvise it among ourselves.

This need was so great in one that he broke down in tears at the impossibility of the enormous task of explaining himself and giving a full account of all that he had done. The need is particularly urgent in a hospital, where you know you are, must be, to some extent, mad. You want to make your story known in order to reconstruct and reclaim the thread of yourself. The feeling of selfhood, under assault from conditions which work by confusing it so chaotically, is trying to buttress itself by trumpeting achievements, starting wild enterprises and seeking recognition from others. This is what psychiatric diagnoses term grandiosity.

It is incredibly hard to hold the words and ideas in, even when you know you cause alarm by talking too fast. The psychoanalyst Darian Leader writes and talks about 'delusions offering solutions', which makes good sense. By pouring all the igniting fires of my ideas and inspirations into a grand narrative, into the thriller in which I am living, I am able to

gain some control of this need to be known in all my variations and to explain myself in all my fracturing details. My
delusions function as a brake, a map and a comforting pattern,
something to hang on to and pursue through the eruptions
of emotion and thought which beset me.

Meanwhile, in the high mountains, my work for my unseen
masters becomes more fun. At dusk I prepare for action at
the head of the valley. The highest peaks are a stone dragon's
face, a brutal, twisted creature, its eyes wide and wild, the
nostrils flaring, the teeth – the peaks running down the valley
– horribly bared. We are all in the dragon's mouth. For a
moment I can see it, I know it. I feel a gut lurch of terror.

The night is freezing and luminous. Rebecca and the boys
have finished skiing and are safe in the hotel. I am free.
Tonight's challenge is a timed race back to the village. I must
be as quick and daring and surreptitious as possible.

Throwing myself down a steep bank, my body is a
toboggan. I cross a snowfield at a racing sprint. Now I am
in the back lanes of a settlement, placing my feet in frozen
footprints. I am climbing fences, ghosting over ice, making
snow angels on a bank, navigating along dark footpaths. I am
on the banks of a wide beck, its water running black. By
fording it I will cut out a long turn in the valley and win the
race. I take off my boots and socks, roll up my jeans and
wade. It is shreddingly cold. My feet burn and I am as happy
as I have ever been, the whole great valley a glowing theatre,
the mountains and the hidden soldiers my audience.
Somewhere, my team, my trainers and supporters, are
cheering me on. On the other side of the beck I hop around
in snow and pine needles, laughing and cursing.

A pristine field might be sown with landmines but a
paddock with horses in it must be safe. Here are electric
fences, here are a car's tracks. Exultant I press on. My goal
is the ski hire shop underneath one of the cable car stations
– the British forces' forward operating base. Once I get there

I am 'home'. I make it in what I feel sure is good time, arriving triumphantly at the Hotel Medil.

You could not design a more wonderful crucible than the Val di Fassa for a madman to act out his fantasies, unknown and mostly unobserved. The great frozen stage feeds my soul, exercising and even exorcising me. But in the morning, in the small hours, we are going home. The world is about to close in.

I am packed: the mattress is propped against the wall (a lunatic's idea of a thorough clean-up). I annoy the bus driver, a less sympathetic person than our driver Alex. He seems quite highly strung. It is 4 a.m.

'What's his problem?' I ask Rebecca, bemused.

'You're late! You're keeping everyone waiting.'

'All right, all right.'

At the next stop, a pick-up from another hotel, it strikes me that I need a cigarette and the bus needs its engine off: we are polluting the whole valley. I switch it off and hop out.

The bus driver goes berserk, shouting in good English with a strong Austrian accent.

'You are a fucking crazy person! What the fuck you think you are doing?'

'The coach driver was at his wits' end,' Rebecca recalls. 'He wanted to batter you. That lovely man Joe and a couple of the other guys who were on the coach got off and they sort of calmed the situation down. Joe took you away because you liked him.

'He came up to me in the queue for check-in – we had all the bags and you'd just fucked off – and Joe came up to me and said, "I think someone needs to give you a medal and I wish I had one, because you deserve one."'

CHAPTER 3

Break-up

Kate, Rebecca's sister, works for the intelligence services. She has recently been promoted. Her official job is a perfect cover – she is a director of strategy for the NHS, so can be anywhere anytime, unavailable for mysterious good reasons, dealing in worlds her friends and family know little about. Fond of fast cars and sarcasm, Kate has a warm, gay disposition. She meets us at Manchester airport and escorts us to her sporty four-by-four. I am suspicious of cars, particularly recent models. It is too easy to be filmed, bugged, tracked and watched in a car like this. I take the front passenger seat, the boys and Rebecca get in the back.

Kate slices through the sleet and traffic, chatting happily, asking the children about the trip. We are all rather quiet, thanks to the 4 a.m start and thanks to me. I am very quiet. I am unsure of where I stand in relation to Kate. I know she is in on it. Will she act as a case officer to me, or does my position in the middle of all this mean she is waiting for my instructions? What has she been told to do? I trust her but not the spooks behind her. I maintain an aggressive silence.

Kate overshoots a motorway turn-off, and says, 'OK, so this is how we do this,' and starts to move swiftly through the traffic, watching all her mirrors closely, before taking the next slip road, flicking around the roundabout and gliding back down into the traffic, now heading back towards the airport. She does the same trick again but this time takes the missed turning off the motorway.

In reality she has simply missed a turning and talked herself through a roundabout, but I assume I am being instructed in counter-surveillance driving and I am annoyed. It is good of Kate to confirm my belief in what is going on, and her role in it, but it is mischievous of her employers to make a play for me like this. They must understand that for the process to work I have to remain independent. Presumably they cannot help trying for an advantage, despite the risk to the negotiations. It means I will have to demonstrate my neutrality again, my integrity and my deep hostility to the absurd nationalist policies which have brought the world to its desperate state.

I know how fortunate I am to hold a British (and European) passport but I prize my mongrel heritage: Welsh, English, Russian. (My father's DNA test showed traces of Indian and Ashkenazi too.) My surname is French: there may be no French blood in me but I feel proudly European. I have adopted France and Sicily, where I have lived, as spiritual homelands, along with Wales. I feel little loyalty to any nation state compared to my commitment to international understanding, to the dream of a world without border walls or frontiers, where humanity works for the common good, for the good of all people and the earth. That is what I am fighting for. This, I presume, is why I have been dragged into all this.

My history of precarious mental health helps to qualify me for my part. The highs and heavy lows I have experienced give me a degree of cover, a kind of ready-made deniability. I am a useful chaotic element: I might 'go off on one', as it were, at any point, meaning that none of the governments or agencies negotiating our future can recruit me, coerce me or wholly rely on me: I cannot be used to load the dice in negotiations. I am a cut-out. No one will ever know what role I played. I will have to suffer, I understand, but that is fine by me.

Kate takes us to Rochdale, to the sisters' family home, where we left my car before we went skiing. I am annoyed with her and Rebecca by now. I want out and away. I no longer want to be with Rebecca. I see her treatment of me on the holiday as a bombardment of dismissal and unkindness. It is time we broke up. I jump out of the car, hop into mine and take off. Rebecca has a car there – she can drive herself home. I am fed up with her. She and Kate call out, trying to stop me, but I ignore them. Above Todmorden, on the way home, I stop at a pub and treat myself to a meal alone and a pint. Having been travelling since 3 a.m UK time, on no sleep, I shouldn't be driving at all, never mind after a drink.

We own a flat in Hebden Bridge. It is small, with a view of roofs and woods, the repository of savings and earnings others might have put in pensions, an investment intended for Robin. I sleep there, on the sofa-bed in the small front room. It is all over with Rebecca, I decide. Tomorrow I will tell her so.

In the morning Kate drives us both to Halifax, to the hospital, where I have agreed to be assessed. I no longer want to be with her but if going to see someone will get her off my back, I am happy to do it. I still mind about her. We are going to have to work out our separation: I will see a doctor, or whoever it is she wants me to see, to mollify her. In the hospital car park I inform Rebecca and Kate that I wish to break up with Rebecca, that we are no longer a couple. I make it clear that I do not wish her to have any role in my care; I do not consent for any of my personal data to be shared with her, and I name a friend of ours, Emma, as my official first point of contact, a kind of unofficial next of kin. I have not warned Emma or asked her if she will accept the appointment. I settle on her off the top of my head, and for no better reason than that she is very clever and dynamic, and not quite as close to our family as some of our other local friends. Thus she is more likely, I believe, to be objective, and less readily influenced by Rebecca.

I am aware that Rebecca and her sister are trying to help but I resent them. I do not trust them. If Kate is compromised by her work for the Security Service then how could Rebecca not be?

During the interview with two women on the crisis team, a psychiatrist and a student, I explain myself as clearly as I can. I tell them I have experienced two crises hitherto: one in 2008, at the culmination of a long journey across Africa; one in 2016, in France. Both involved stress, heat, exhaustion and cannabis. In France I saw two doctors, who diagnosed cyclothymia, a mild form of bipolar. The French doctors told me that the condition is manageable, with sleep, food, good relationships and a careful avoidance of narcotics and stress. (Cyclothymia does not seem to have gained much traction with the British medical establishment.)

The psychiatrist and the student listen sympathetically as I confess that I have fallen off the wagon, using cannabis and alcohol to excess, and that there are problems and stresses at home. I tell them I do not require medication.

'I was prescribed loxapine by the doctor in France who diagnosed cyclothymia,' I say. 'She advised me to take it if I found myself behaving in a manic way – not sleeping, and talking too fast.'

All the while I am holding a copy of *The Light in the Dark*, a book I wrote about winter and seasonal depression. I have brought it with me in order to convince myself and the doctors that I am a serious person who has thought about what I am saying. It works. The psychiatrist seems tentatively satisfied. I agree to stay in contact with the crisis team. I can talk to them daily on the phone, they say, and they would like me to receive visits over the Christmas period to check

that I am OK. I say that is fine by me. They ask me to enter
a self-administered alcohol- and drug-reduction programme,
to which I agree. I ask them to assess Rebecca as well, for
stress – she surely needs support. Rebecca goes in to talk to
them after me. Her session went like this:

'The psychiatrist said that they felt that there was something that didn't ring true about your story, that it was just
that you were drinking lots and taking drugs – it didn't seem
like you were a habitual drug-taker or drinker. But because
you kept saying we've split up, I don't want her to have access
to my data or anything, and that you were happy to do whatever they thought you needed to do, they said, "There's
nothing we can do if you're not living together." I said, "I'm
here with my sister, we've just come back from a skiing
holiday, we've been together for eleven years." They said,
"No no no, he's saying that his mother is the next of kin."
The crisis team can't do anything if you're not willing to
engage with them, which you weren't.'

There is no easy way to perform the hellish role that falls
on those who are closest to the chaotically distressed.
Somehow Rebecca opens and maintains lines of communication with my family (who are miles away) and closest friends,
and her family. She looks after our son. It is the school
holidays, so she arranges a full programme of events, days
with his friends, with her family, expeditions with her and
others. She does not neglect her own care, talking on the
phone to a counsellor provided by her employers and keeping
up her regular running schedule. She does whatever she can
for me, resistant though I am. She spends hours navigating
the health service's systems, trying to establish what care
might be available and how best to access it.

There is a serious and desperate difference in access to
health services for those living in poorer and richer areas – a
difference exemplified by Rebecca. Highly educated, with a
broad span of connections (including her NHS strategist

sister), naturally inquisitive and a sophisticated communicator, she is superbly placed to discover and access available services. And yet when we talk about this dreadful time afterwards, what emerges is that her ceaseless efforts met with repeated frustration.

'As far as I was concerned the crisis team were rubbish all the way through,' she says. 'The police were wonderful. What people have to know about this situation is that if you're supporting someone who is having a breakdown you have to be strong and stick to it, you have to keep asking for help, you have to not be fobbed off by them saying, "Oh, it's just drink and drugs." If it's not, if it's more than that, then you have to get the support of your friends and family around you and provide support. You can't be gaslit by someone saying "It doesn't sound like they are a danger to themselves or others" and making you think you're in the wrong. If they are a danger to themselves you have to say it and keep saying it. The system doesn't work.'

CHAPTER 4

Manic Christmas

It is early morning. I went to bed late last night but I snap awake. I am looking forward to everything, to the hot dousing of the shower, to the taste and dark jolt of coffee, to the blush of nicotine from my first cigarette, to the smell of the new day, to the emails, to the work, to the next project (and all those unfinished schemes), to the first drink (which I will probably have around lunchtime), to everything, everything.

It is as though I am permanently coming up on Ecstasy. Today is one of the best of my life. No encounter will be without significance. Along with my optimism and my hunger for the full taste of every moment, I have a raging sex drive. I will entertain a thousand fantasies. I will flirt with everyone.

Today I have left the flat. I am now alone in the family house; Rebecca has taken our son away to stay with her ex-husband and his family. It is for the best that we are separated. Everything is for the best. It is Christmas Eve and I have done as much as I can. Last night I went to Rochdale, where her family live, and abandoned my car outside her ex-husband's house with a scrawled note and all sorts of presents for him and his family: magnets, clockwork fish, books, electronic things, something for all of them, unwrapped and scattered like shining junk across the seats and boot.

Before that I went to a pub, the Baum, and ran into old friends. There was Alastair who used to run a fire station in

Australia (I am sure he does covert work for the armed forces now) and, in the garden behind the pub, Bushra, who introduced me to a glittering young woman who I worked out was part of the Moroccan royal family, who seemed to approve of me.

No doubt the secret negotiations have reached a vital stage – the liberal Islam of Morocco has long been a preoccupation of mine, and I want the kingdom to reform, since I met those dissidents in Italy last month and they told me that the price of bread has gone up tenfold, and the repression increased, and the king has been prevented by incompetent politicians from helping his people, and dozens of overlapping secret services are fighting for power, and the king's modern and brilliant young wife, who gave such hope to the population, has separated from him and withdrawn.

And so I pledged my support to the young woman and talked and drank and smoked and hauled presents and finally took a taxi home. I am obsessed with Islam now, and find myself in many debates and discussions with taxi drivers, men knowledgeable and concerned about their faith.

In the taxi back from Rochdale I took the role of student to an elderly gentleman who carried himself with great dignity, who gave his pronouncements the force of grave import.

'When the second coming of Jesus comes,' he told me, 'Jesus will announce that he is a Muslim. Many people will turn against him and they will not be saved. You will only be saved if you swear to be loyal to him, if you have never said anything against Muhammad, peace be upon him, and if you can cross into paradise over a bridge which is as narrow as a needle.'

I hoard this knowledge, this truth.

After Christmas, I will tip taxi drivers fistfuls of notes. Bewildered, they will try to give the money back but I will not take it, leaving it on the seat and running away. I believe the money will be taken as a tribute to Islam. I believe that giving it away is a contribution to the understanding between cultures. Throughout the mania, money accrues increasing symbolic worth, as its actual value becomes insignificant. An entire value system of tribute and sharing will dominate my daily practice, my rituals and my fantasy.

Anyway, this evening, Christmas Eve, I am due at my friend Doug's house. But first, a support worker is coming from the crisis team to see how I am getting on with my drug- and alcohol-reduction programme and my exercise plan. I am reducing my intake of intoxicants but only minutely, which means I still have a spicy rollie, flecking it with tiny spots of sweet resin, as well as a shot of rum in my coffee, because it's Christmas.

Now something strange happens. I find myself in some part of the Internet I do not know and a chat window opens, requesting a security code. From something I was sent or obtained, I have a code, and enter it. Now another black window opens; the mic is live on the laptop and I find myself speaking with someone in America. He sounds alert, intelligent, somewhat frayed – he sounds like someone with whom I would get along. He seems to be on a conference call with someone else.

'Are you there?' he asks, speaking to me, it seems. I say I am.

'How's it going?'

'Not bad,' I say. 'How is it with you?'

'Well we're all just running to keep up here,' he says.

It is late morning with me, so I presume he is on the East Coast, up early. The accent is educated, the speech rapid and articulate. We could be on a current-affairs programme; I half expect him to deliver a report.

'The fact is, there is no protocol for this situation,' he says.

'What situation?'

'First contact,' he says seriously, and we both laugh.

'But it's going well?'

'I think so,' he says. 'It's quite confused. And you're OK over there?'

'I think so,' I reply.

Not long afterwards we bid each other farewell. I have the impression that both of us understood that the call was not private, that we had to be careful with what we said. We were both excited and cautious.

I am in no doubt. First contact! For Christ's sake – *it is all real*! You can't get closer to final confirmation than that, I think exultantly. (In this, too, I am wrong.)

The support worker turns up exactly on time. She is beautiful. I settle her on the sofa with tea and flirt gently with her, sympathising with her workload over Christmas, apologising for being part of it.

'Exercise is going well! I'm doing lots. I walk everywhere or take my bike.'

I do too. I have been cycling like a maniac. I have been pounding on foot through the woods and charging downhill at a sprint: I wiped out a couple of days ago; I was lucky to break no bones. I leave that out.

I am honest about reducing the dope and booze but vague about the quantities. I love them both and I am not going to stop. The bike is equipped with a transmitter which allows the security services to track you. It is a flashy machine. I came by it apparently by mistake in Cambridge, when I was there for the literary festival a couple of weeks ago. I was trying to buy dope from a wildly paranoid street dealer. He took my forty pounds, leaving me with a mountain bike (which I assume he had stolen) as security. When he did not come back I loaded the bike into the car, assuming it was a clever ruse by the security services to pass me special equipment.

I do not tell her that. And I do not care about the tracker. There is a kind of paranoia that does not resent the forces it assumes are working unseen: you accept being of special interest because after all you are special. Your mind and imagination are working hectically to put a wall of confidence and significance between you and the facts.

A psychotic middle-aged man whose behaviour has estranged him from his family, who now faces Christmas alone? You would laugh, genuinely bemused, at the suggestion that this is you.

The support worker leaves and I go about my hectic business. There is still more to buy. I have been told I am not welcome at the family Christmas lunch in Rochdale but I have insisted I will go over in the morning anyway, to give out presents.

As night falls I go to Doug's house. He takes me up to his study and plays a trick on me, flicking a spot of water at me while doing a sleight of hand with a plastic severed thumb.

'OK,' he says, as he does it. 'This is it.'

In reality it is only a little practical joke, but the move shakes me deep down. So this is how they do it. Finally, the secret ceremony. I have been ordained into MI6. My friend Doug will be my controller – or that is what they want. I am flattered, thrilled, slightly scared and slightly resentful. Won't this prejudice the negotiations? Doug's father is here, a lovely man, a former teacher at a private school. Obviously he has long been a recruiter for the service, and here he is, welcoming me aboard. A programme I made with Radio 3 back in the autumn, before I was manic, is transmitting now. Doug has it on in the kitchen. It is strange to hear it, edited and ordered, a reminder that anyone can be portrayed any way. Be careful. Rebecca is here too, having brought our son over from Rochdale for the carol singing, a tradition she loves, so I flick some water at her. We are all in this together, at last.

'Here, have this, it will keep you warm,' says Doug, presenting me with a red fleecy body warmer. It is Parachute-Regiment red. Be careful.

Every Christmas Eve the whole town gathers in the square to sing carols around the tree. It is a beautiful tradition and I have written about it in the book which I am currently promoting. It makes me very self-conscious as I circle the crowd. A lot of them seem to be looking at me. What do they know? What do they think? I keep my distance from my family, just in case.

Back up the hill, outside Doug's house again, I stand with Phil, another friend – Phil with his brilliant mind, his tendency to mild mania, his baby strapped across his chest under his jacket, and his T-shirt para red.

All of a sudden I realise what is going on. Out here, in Doug's garden on the edge of the wood, I could be shot down from a dozen directions.

Phil is asking me questions about my relationship, about where I am in my head, about how I am. Oh God. This is it. They are going to execute me, with Phil standing right there, as in those live-fire exercises the SAS practise. Cold certain fear grips my stomach and floods down my legs. I am as scared as I have ever been. Will it hurt, when the bullet strikes? How will they arrange it? They can fix anything. What will they tell my son – that I was mad? That I shot myself? A pistol planted by my body? Will it be said that they killed me to prevent a rampage?

'You OK?'

'I'm not sure. I just . . .'

'Wait a second,' Phil says. 'This is all wrong.'

He means the set-up, the plan for my execution. But does he have the authority to stop it?

I make it back into Doug's house, and later, somehow, home, after a jinking tour through the town, where I stick to the shadows and pop up in random bars. Every time I approach a bar I go through a rapid and conscientious ritual, turning out all my pockets. Here are mini-screwdrivers, euro coins, playing cards, nails, talismanic bits of Lego, glitterings of odds and ends I have picked off pavements.

Each time I stand at a bar I get it all out, spread it all in plain sight. It all means something to the watchers. I am saying, by gesture, over and over, I am me, I have nothing to hide. Here is my heart. Here are all my signs.

I am one flickered look from getting beaten up in the White Swan by a young man as wild as me who shouts in my face, 'There's something up with this guy. Hey! I don't like you. I don't fucking like you. I'll fucking smack you . . .'

Another odd person, a huge man dressed in shamanic robes and a flamboyant hat, befriends me at the bar. He is on drugs, fizzing with them. We grin and bristle at each in a fight-or-flight circling, then a coming-together. Eight, nine, ten months later people I half-recognise will greet me, remembering some seemingly deep and instant connection made briefly now.

Christmas Day. I am allowed to see Rebecca and the family in Rochdale but I am expected to leave before Christmas lunch. Her parents and sister hover around me as I write cards to uncles and aunts at their dining table. This must be the worst Christmas of their lives. I am entirely oblivious to it.

My son is playing uncertainly with his new toys. His grandfather, Rebecca's father, stands behind me at one point, holding a kitchen knife. It suddenly occurs to me that he must be a Mason, that this may be some sort of initiation moment. I tilt my head back, baring my throat.

Upstairs Rebecca's nephew is playing Fortnite. I look into his room in time to see him put two bullets into the back of a man wearing a white shirt. I assume this is a message for me. A little later I am sitting on the stairs, arguing with Rebecca. 'Marry me or fuck off!' I shout.

Rebecca and Kate herd me out. I drive back to Hebden. I am expected at a Christmas meal in town, with friends, neighbours of Doug's. I manage half an hour of it, eating a plateful of the main course, before lurching off again.

I have a very short temper now, caused by a combination of the irritability of the high, the bone-deep exhaustion which I refuse to acknowledge, and frustration with the way people who love me look at me, react to me, speak to me. It is much easier to be with strangers. The cordial codes of meeting and exchanging pleasantries that guide new encounters protect both sides. Being around those who know me is almost impossible, but there are still one or two I trust, and who can take me. One is Zaffar Kunial, poet. On Boxing Day night we go for a drink.

In the Old Gate pub we choose our beer, then I take us outside so that I can smoke. There is an electric cold in the air. It seems to jump through me.

'How's Rebecca?' Zaff asks gently, 'I heard you guys . . .'

'It's been tough but it's the right thing you know, much better. She's fine, I mean she's not fine but you know what I mean. The main thing is the boys, but it's going to be fine. It's . . . hard . . . How are you?'

'Yeah not bad! OK. So – are you – do you want to talk about it?'

'Yes I'm fine talking about it. It's really lovely to see you actually, I've missed you! How are you? What have you been reading?'

Now I am messing about with my car, which is parked outside the pub. The seats and footwells are a chaos of books and presents and clothes.

'Jump in, Zaff! Let's go for a drive. I'm going to Wales tonight, to my Mum's. I'm on my way actually but I'd like to just check on the house, make sure they're all tucked up. We won't go and bother them, we can see from the other side of the valley, the road through the wood.'

'You're going tonight?' He looks at the diminishing pint in my hand. 'Are you sure you're OK to drive?'

'Yes yes! I've only had this. I'm good to go.'

'Are you quite sure? You could go tomorrow.'

'It's better at night. It's a really good time. The roads will
be empty. I've been thinking about Shakespeare a lot.
Definitely need some woods . . .'

Zaff climbs in and we go slowly up the hill towards
Heptonstall and follow the lane through the woods. Last year
we drove to Hay together, one hot summer day, talking about
poetry and writing, about our parents and our lives all the
long green way. The happiness and curiosity and delight in
his company that I felt then I feel now. I wish Zaff was
coming with me, I wish we could drive again to Wales and
that everything could be as it was. By talking with him about
books and travels I feel I can almost recapture it. But this
drive is too short, too peculiar to give us more than an echo.

We nose along a narrow lane which overlooks our valley.
Just across from us, on the other side, we can see my house.
The lights shine through tangled black trees. Rebecca and
the children are safe inside.

'Oh look! The attic light is on. I'll just tell her. Can I
borrow your phone?'

Zaff waits while I get out and make the call. I try a forced
brightness, a sort of sing-song: 'Hi love! How are you? Just
calling to say the light in the attic is on!'

Rebecca is alarmed and hostile. I cannot understand why.
I am rude. I hang up.

Brusque now, finding it harder to cast our situation as
cheerful, I turn the car in the lane. Zaff has become quieter.

'Take care,' he says when I drop him in town.

'You too, dear Zaff! Happy Christmas,' I cry, hugging
him, overlooking the fact that Christmas has passed and Zaff
does not celebrate it. I set the car south and west for Wales,
for home.

CHAPTER 5

A goshawk and Kylie Minogue

I love long night drives, the service stations, the empty roads, even the motorway coffee. This time I buy an audio book, *A Possible Life* by Sebastian Faulks, read by Samuel West. Somewhere north of Birmingham the traffic is filtered into a single lane. Lines of lorries queue like pack animals. The audio book begins to behave strangely, West's beautiful voice chanting like a psalm, seeming to address me directly.

I realise that the audio has been hijacked by the controlling forces. I have been wondering when I would hear from them again. Following the words and rhythms of the voice, I change lanes and vary my speed. Fortunately we are all travelling slowly. I guess I am being instructed in the art of guided driving: no doubt drones and cameras are being deployed as part of the exercise. West's instructions take me off the motorway into a deserted and unknown country, the roads as still as if they had never been driven, houses as dark as if they had never been occupied. By the time I find myself in Church Stretton, in Shropshire, it is very late.

My grandmother lived here. The last time I saw her was in her garden, just down the road there. Granny had an absolute certainty about who she was and what she wanted. Her memory is reassuring. I pull up in a supermarket car park, the nearest place to her house I can find somewhere to stop. Under the white glare of a security light I wind back my seat and sleep.

Before dawn I wake and join another stream of southbound lorries, arriving home in the early morning. There is my mother, excited to have her boys back – my brother will be coming later – and there is the farm, and the dog. Here is my childhood home, my safest place, eternal in the frost.

My brother is coming home tonight. I am very excited and my mother is too. He has been in America. He has an influential job with a big company – although he is in public relations we do not really know what he has been doing. I know he has done work for the aerospace industry and I suspect he has been drawn into the realms of defence and security. I assume he will be in contact with significant players in the great enterprise (he is very keen on his phone), and although I am wary of whatever his agenda may be, I love him and cannot wait to see him.

He comes in late, shaking hands, grinning, bringing cheer. He has turned himself into a film-maker – his first short film has recently been premiered at a New York festival. I am under the impression that he has had something to do with what is on television at the moment, which turns out to be a programme about Kylie Minogue. The programme has her sitting in a cinema with the presenter, watching and commenting on clips from her career.

'Watch it, H!' my brother says.

I do. I can't believe it. Now that I am separated from Rebecca I am on the lookout for a new relationship. I understand that, given my precarious place in the great enterprise, any relationship I might form will be subject to huge scrutiny. I suspect the people in charge of the secret negotiations will have strong feelings about who I am allowed to see, about who might be allowed to get close to me – but here is the most extraordinary result. Kylie Minogue!

It's insane. It's ludicrous! It's wonderful. She must have been involved in all this for much longer than me. Of course, she is exactly the sort of cultural ambassador you would want as part of a worldwide peace process. And, of course, I have adored her since the 1980s. We must be nearly the same age. God knows I've danced to enough of her songs. And here she is, looking at me!

The programme I am watching has her staring at the camera as if at the screen on which she is watching clips of her concerts and videos, so she stares out at me with a mixture of amusement, conspiracy, embarrassment and even delight, like those moments in *Blind Date* when the screen went back.

'I'm going to marry Kylie Minogue!' I announce. And I mean it.

It's a lot to think about, but I must not neglect my duties.

The next day I go into town with my mother. There is a rug sale on in the Clarence Hall in Crickhowell. My mother knows the merchant and does not particularly trust him, but I have a feeling that I need to engage with him: he is another bridge between cultures. He is a bluff, loquacious salesman with quick eyes and a self-conscious, harried manner. His assistant is a stocky and watchful younger man, obviously in the military. I circle the rugs and settle on one.

'It's eight hundred pounds. I can take six by cheque and two in cash?'

'I'm not sure I can do that.'

'I really need to take the six now, and it will make a huge difference if you can do the two?'

The salesman and his assistant are looking at me almost pleadingly. I cannot afford this carpet, but the urgency of the situation speaks of its wider importance. I am being asked to demonstrate commitment and good faith. This is a symbolic trade of potentially vast impact – these carpets come from Afghanistan, from Iran, from countries where we have done enormous damage, nations to which we must make redress and pay respect. My petty cash problems are as nothing in comparison to such a demonstration of good faith. Of course I must do my part, unhesitatingly, generously, immediately. No doubt it will all balance out in the end. God knows I am working hard enough for the great cause. I am certain the government will reimburse me at some point, by some subtle means.

'Ok, done,' I say, and produce my card, and go to the cash point, and hand it all over to the delighted salesman. His soldier takes the carpet to my car. He seems very respectful. I have a feeling that I have made a good and important decision, some payment of compensation, perhaps, to families which were harmed by Western action in Afghanistan.

My mother is unimpressed. It's not a very special carpet, Turkish, she thinks, and significantly overpriced. I can see her point but I am sure there are greater forces at play. I am not sure how much Mum knows about what is going on. There are (actual) former spies among her old friends. Another former spy bought our last house. I know she once asked her friend in MI6 for a job.

'He said, but you wouldn't be prepared to sleep with people, would you?' and I said, "No!" and he said well there you are then,' as she tells it.

But who knows what really went on? Mum is a dynamite student of human nature. I can imagine her as an interrogator or as a wise consultant. She is extremely well informed on world events, listening to Radio 4 much of the day and the World Service much of the night. She seems sanguine about the purchase, overall; her way of dealing with me when I am high is to tell me I am, to advise me not to drink, to feed me, to maintain a hopeful and open dialogue, while urging me to seek treatment.

My brother is more stressed by my behaviour, or less able to control stress, though I can see him battling to let me be, to let me babble and relax. He cares for me very much. I am trying not to upset him by talking too much and too fast. We go for a walk in the afternoon. He talks about Elon Musk and electric vehicles.

'One problem is they are so quiet they are dangerous,' he says.

Immediately I understand. He has said before that he is a fan of Musk. He has been working with him, no doubt. And they are stuck on this problem of noise, and they are asking me for help. Right!

I have picked up a broken shard of bone, a sheep's foreleg. Now I drag it along the tarmac of the lane.

'How about this? Perfect, no? Not too loud, but you can definitely hear it!'

Alexander looks at me strangely. While he fights not to be upset by my behaviour or angered by my resistance to going to the doctor, I fight not to allow my mania to rush out and provoke him.

We are having an argument in the kitchen about whether I should see a doctor.

'You were saying you're going to marry Kylie Minogue! You were dragging a broken bone along the road!'

'Oh come on! You asked me what I thought and I told you – that's completely unfair!'

'Well,' my mother butts in. 'You are rather high, and we are worried. What's the harm in going to Brecon and seeing a doctor? I've rung and there is someone you can see.'

'Because I don't need to. I've told you – I'm ringing up the crisis team in Calderdale every day, I'm in an alcohol and drugs reduction programme, I'm seasonally affective and I'm taking vitamin D – there's nothing more anyone can do.'

'There's no need to shout. We'll just go, just to reassure me and your brother then – why not?'

'Oh, OK then. But are you really going to drive?'

'Of course! You are so rude about my driving.'

Mum drives us perfectly to Brecon. At the health centre I see a doctor from Shropdoc, a not-for-profit company providing out-of-hours care across a swathe of Shropshire and Powys, available through the NHS on 111. I trot out my usual refrain. Cynically, I point out that my brother, as I see it, has anger management issues. He becomes angry. The doctor listens to me, to my brother, to my mother. Mum is caught. She is very conscious of being my 'nearest relative'. She wants me to have help but she keeps promising me that nobody is going to take me away. She finds herself arguing both sides.

'He is high, yes, but he's not dangerous,' she tells the doctor.

The doctor offers sedatives. He is clearly unhappy about the situation, but since I am not apparently dangerous . . . I take one to please them. Home we go. I am back in control, I decide. If we are a unit, I am the senior officer, Mum is my lieutenant, and my brother a slightly rogue junior officer. In the morning I am as normal, in my eyes, and as manic, in theirs, as I was the day before.

My brother tries to have a normal time. He watches films until late, as he does, and sleeps late, and eats our traditional big breakfasts, and reads and goes for walks.

My mother feeds the sheep and looks after the farm. I help her when required. At night I sit with candles in the kitchen, which alarms my mother. She does not trust me not to set fire to the house. I am involved in another crisis – a rift between my brother and our father. For much of their dispute I have tried to act as a go-between, pushing them towards each other, passing news of their doings and asking-afterings from one to the other. But now I am impatient and upset with them. I tell them to sort it out themselves.

'How is your brother?' Dad asks on the phone.

In a tone as coldly hostile as I have ever used with him, I reply, 'Have you asked him?'

Dad sounds shocked, but he rides it. 'I see,' he says. He is actually seriously ill, but I am beginning to suspect the hospital might have mistaken or manipulated his test results. I expect he is getting better.

Underneath so much of it, this.

Now comes the New Year, and a rush of activity, hidden and overt, on the world's stages. One of my mother's highlights of the year is the *Correspondents' Look Ahead*, a Radio 4 programme which brings together eminent journalists and asks them for their thoughts on the countries they cover and their predictions for the year ahead. Mum loves the programme. This year I am duty-bound to listen to it carefully too, for I am sure my views will be sought and tested.

The night of the programme I am operating on my toe. Ever since I kicked the bed in the Hotel Medil the big toe of my right foot has been angry-red and mildly infected. I have lost the nail; the whole toe is painful and swollen. I retrieve the medicine tin from the bathroom, set up with needle, antiseptic, dressing and a candle flame, and prepare to operate. My brother is horrified and offended. 'What are you doing? Operating on yourself? This is mad. Go to the doctor!'

'I don't need a doctor. It's simple first aid.'

Furious and despairing, he withdraws.

I swab the toe with antiseptic, heat the needle until it glows red, then jab it into the most swollen parts of my toe. There is some egress of pus, not the satisfying dam-burst I was hoping for, but something. I dress my toe and plan to do the same thing tomorrow, or whenever it swells up again. With hindsight it seems fairly characteristic behaviour – I am keen on first aid – but my enthusiasm for carrying out painful procedures on myself was not a healthy impulse, and it began to grow.

I have to prove I am fit, resolute, prepared to shed blood and spend money in the service of a greater cause, that is the thing. Looking no further back than the last few days, with their freight of the last few weeks, there seems to be a powerful and simple motor beneath the mania. I am seeking and creating adventure and challenge because I am in grief at the separation from my family and in guilt for the way I am behaving. Clearly, some part of me knows this, but the rest of me is working hard to keep that perception submerged, foundering under tides of action and fantasy. Mania and psychosis spin through fury, hilarity, glee, paranoia and arousal. They leave no room for grief or guilt.

New Year's Eve, the Farmers Arms, Cwmdu. Men I have known since we were boys are dancing and singing. My brother and I are at the bar. I am talking to him, and to a woman, a friend of the owners, and to her partner, who is as vivid and wild as I am – he tells a story of taking mushrooms recently and finding himself standing on a table, naked and roaring – and I am hearing and mishearing snatches of conversation from all sides.

I am putting it all together in my head in a carnivalesque fantasy. The wild man I believe to be D. B. C. Pierre, the writer. I think he is trying to tell me that he is an illegitimate child of my father's, that we are half-brothers. I am shocked and sorry that we did not meet before, that our childhoods were spent on opposite sides of the world, but I am delighted that we have met now.

At the same time I am hearing from the dancing farmers that someone we know and like is secretly a terrible person, guilty of fearful crimes, and that they are waiting for my approval for a plan they have to kill him: they are going to blow the tyres on his four-by-four as he drives the twisting road from Bwlch; he will be killed in the crash. They are quite sure of his guilt but they want me to sanction his assassination. I drink. I am appalled at the thought of it, at the revelation that this quiet Welsh world can be conceal such evil. I am sick with a kind of horrified grief that our friend is so dangerous and cruel. It can't be. It *can't* be. But it is. It will be done. The moral responsibility for the action is on me.

Later, Alexander and Mum asleep, I am awake in the kitchen, listening to the news on the World Service. I chip in when it seems apposite, giving approval to hints I believe the reporters are giving me. This person will rise, this person will fall. Benevolent world government which takes account of the observations of journalists seems a good system, though it is exhausting to be part of it all. I imagine terrible demonstrations of alien power – American and Chinese embassies destroyed by weapons of unearthly might; I can foresee it, I can almost hear the screams. I can almost feel the world coming together. I can almost see a new and beautiful planet being born out of the fires which surround us.

My mother will not let me go home until I have been to the doctor's in Crickhowell. She has hidden my car keys. Eventually she agrees that as long as I register with a local doctor, so that I can access treatment if and when I return to Wales, she will give me back my keys.

'Fine, I'll go. But I'm walking.'

I am fed up of being driven around like a patient. In the crux between cooperating in my own care and retaining a sense of agency and self-directed control, I am beginning seriously to tire of being treated as ill, as other, as abnormal. On a calm winter afternoon, I set out to walk to Crickhowell by a new route, a more-or-less straight line, over the shoulder of the mountain, along the hill fence, down into the back of the town.

Considering that I am going to be married to Kylie Minogue, that last night I took moral responsibility for the murder of a friend who had turned out to be a terrible perpetrator of crimes, and given that I am engaged in a secret worldwide effort to bring about universal change, on pain of planetary destruction by aliens, I feel meditative and peaceful as I walk. Above the village, on the lower slopes of the mountain which overlooks Cwmdu, I meet one of our neighbours, a farmer who is a good friend to my mother. He has evidently been drinking milk from a large bottle; there is a ring of white smear around his mouth.

'Hello there!'

'All right there? Going for a walk, is it?'

'Yes, I'm going to go along the hills to Crickhowell.'

'How's your mother then?'

'She's well, thank you. How are things with you?'

And all the while, as we talk, I am looking at the ring of milk around his mouth and realising, with something like horror, what he is signalling to me. *We suckled at the same breast.* He is my mother's son. We are half-brothers. Jesus Christ! I am shocked to the pit of my stomach but somehow, in some awful way, unsurprised. My parents moved here at the end of the 60s. Who knows what they got up to? Orgies, infidelities, free love? Christ. And this is my brother. He does look a little like me. We have the same frame, similar blond hair. And Mum does care for him very much. He is a lovely man. But really, fuck's sake! My first book told the story of my parents buying the farm, and the collapse of their marriage, and my childhood on the mountain. How wildly, hopelessly, did I miss the true story, then? What a *fool*. I say goodbye to my secret brother and stride on up the hill. Good God . . .

I take bearings on trees and ridges and march south-westwards towards Crickhowell. I move along the field boundaries, cross the fence lines carefully, letting the ground show me where the old lines ran, putting my feet in the prints of centuries. The valley and the hills unfold in new perspectives, aslant. There are buzzards and ravens, jays and magpies, flocks of incurious sheep. I gain the hill fence and cross it, following a contour across waves of ridges and gullies. It is a still, tranquil afternoon of dead bracken under silvery quilts of sky. Now I come down to a hidden valley, deep in the mountain's flank, the slopes towering on either side and a stream falling steeply from the heights. Down towards a larch wood I go, and freeze. There on a branch in front of me, just there, is a goshawk. He perches like a winter emperor on his branch, staring at me with golden eyes.

I sink to my knees, not wanting to scare him, paying him an obeisance, moved by wonder and gratitude. I have never seen one around here, never seen one so close. He has a presence like a messenger from the gods, the old gods below the ground and above the sky, this little centurion, this master of the mountains, the woods, the most secret places. There is an utterness about him, a completeness of shape, strength and marking – he is compounded might and beauty.

For a long time after he flies I remain crouched. Uniquely for this whole long and lonely period of fantasy and derangement, this is an encounter to which I ascribe no mystic significance beyond itself. The goshawk is a marvel, a privilege to encounter, and only that.

Further on, crossing rough ground, I lie back on a fallen tree and stare up at winter's underbelly of hard sky. I can see the motes and scratches on my retinas. It is as though I can see anything and through anything. The power comes with a frightening price, a hypersensitivity, as though the sheaths have peeled off my wiring. I walk under a power line very carefully, scared the current might jump.

The rest of the walk, the visit to the doctor's, registering as a temporary patient, another night of listening to the radio, staying off booze long enough to convince my mother to return my car keys, loading the car and setting off are all accomplished easily. I am calm again, reassured by an encounter in a local hotel where I went to use the Wi-Fi.

The Gliffaes Hotel is a discreetly luxurious Italianate villa set above the River Usk. I worked my first jobs there, washing up and waiting on tables. In the bar there were only two guests, a couple from London in their mid-thirties. They were strikingly beautiful. Chris was tall and heroic-looking, like an army officer from an elite regiment (which I took him to be). Natasha was extremely pretty and even cleverer, perhaps, than her man, whom she said was brilliant.

'We both work for Google,' they said.

We all accepted the fiction.

We talked and shared a joint and bought each other whiskies. They were scared of the coming of the robots and AI. 'They are coming,' they said, 'they are really coming,' and worried about other aspects of their work.

Chris was concerned about quantum computing, and about hypersonic travel.

'The problem is that when you fire an object into space it is only subject to huge temperatures for a short while, passing the atmosphere. But if you fire it around the earth, through the atmosphere, you are heating it up for much longer. And that causes changes to the metals; you can't predict how it's going to go, basically,' Chris said.

I was clear that we were all talking about the UFOs which had been menacing Gatwick, and no doubt other nations' cities and facilities. We were talking about the whole Great Game, at last, as openly as we could. I felt so grateful and so vindicated. How wonderful that these two had been sent to meet me, two obviously decent, brilliant and beautiful people. I was humbled and delighted.

Natasha and Chris were wonderful together – they could not keep their hands off each other, though they tried to, for decorum's sake, which was very sweet to witness. We went out again into the cold to smoke. 'I work for one, two, three, four,' Natasha said, and wordlessly we all think *five*, MI5.

So, the SAS in Chris and the Security Service in her. Good for them for being so direct, at last. 'Departments,' she said, 'and that's where I met this one.' She hugged Chris and shivered. He squeezed her tight and rubbed her arms.

I sensed that they wanted something from me, now that we had exchanged thoughts and met in friendship. We were obviously on the same side.

'There's just so much going on,' Natasha said. 'Don't you find it stressful? It feels like the end of days sometimes.'

'It's going to be fine,' I said. 'What's happening is scary, but it will be OK.'

'But what is it? How do you know?' asked Chris.

'I think it's a revolution in consciousness,' I answered, and as I said it I believed from the bottom of my heart that this was true.

That was what was happening here. If humanity could show itself capable of unity – which after all is really only a question of a bit of horse-trading among politicians, compensation and a UN constitution – then we would get the answers to the technological questions Chris and Natasha were wrestling with. (I was sure our extraterrestrial friends would help with this.) Finally the people of the earth would achieve non-verbal communication, perfect communication: mind-to-mind communion without the disruptions and dislocations of language.

Everything would be different. The revolution would succeed, an uprising in which we would all be victors. *That* was what all this was for.

Chris and Natasha look thoughtful, if not entirely convinced.

'You both call each other "this one",' I observed, grinning at them.

They laughed gleefully.

'I hadn't noticed!' Natasha said.

'I'm sure your friends must have asked you this before,' I said to Chris, 'but . . . have you asked her to marry you?'

He looked at Natasha, adoring and surprised, and his look was reflected in her, and they shouted with laughter and delight, looking rather amazed.

'No one has said that!'

They threw their arms around each other again.

The mad do have that role, after all. We say the obviously unsaid.

They asked about the area, about things to do.

'There's a lovely walk by the river. At the bottom of the steps there's a coracle hut. If you go down the river along the path there's a great walk to Crickhowell . . .'

We parted on the warmest terms. They asked what my plans were.

'I'm going to drive north tomorrow. What's your plan?'

They looked at each other in complete agreement, the handsome man from the SAS and the beautiful girl from MI5.

'We're going to stay in bed,' they said.

CHAPTER 6

Mad at twilight, sane at sunrise

The next morning I turn the car north-west and set off deeper into Wales. I have nothing to hurry back for. My boy is fine; his mother is fine. I am dimly aware that not seeing me must be less stressful than my presence. I will meander my way up. I have a long-held ambition to travel all the roads of this infinite little country. Soon I am lost somewhere in the riddle of mid-Wales, cruising the lanes through the short light of the new year. I stay away from the radio and its threat of mixed messages, listening to music and the engine.

As twilight comes I am high on a ridge, approaching a turning set about with large and urgent signs. I stop and get out. A Ministry of Defence firing range. Danger. Unexploded ordnance. Firing times. Forbidden areas and limited access; safe paths and timings. I struggle to take it all in. There is nothing methodical about my ability to process information at the moment. But the gates are open. This is a safe time, apparently.

The radio is talking to me again. I feel urged to drive onto the range, to park and leave the car.

The car has been worrying me for a while now, with the way the radio started to behave strangely on the way down; the way Sam West's voice was so easily appropriated to give me driving instructions. I know the vehicle is hacked and tracked. Now I have a feeling that the people who know about me are going to do something spectacular with it. I see a fighter jet coming in low and fast, a bomb tumbling through the dusk, the explosion, the crater where the car used to be.

I park on a deserted stretch of road, leave the headlights and hazard lights on and walk away, trying not to run. After three hundred metres I pause and turn. The car sits in the silence, blinking its lights. The last of the sun sinks behind hills. The sunset, the car and a distant house gaudy with Christmas lights are neatly aligned. It will be an easy run for the pilot. I wait for a while. The car flashes forlornly. The cold sharpens. Nothing happens. I shiver and go back, hoping I am not about to be bombed from the air. Eventually I reclaim the driver's seat, turn off the hazard lights and drive away. False alarm. Perhaps it is all over. Perhaps the world's governments have reached an agreement. Perhaps even now the watchers of radar screens are witnessing the departure of alien craft. Perhaps all is well.

A little further on is an unlikely-seeming golf club. What is a golf club doing out here, in the back of beyond? I turn in. I sense something significant. There is a driving range; the lights are on. The radio seems encouraging. Go on, see what's there, it seems to be saying. I jump out and advance.

A stocky, surly man says they are closed to non-members.

'May I look around?'

He shrugs.

Now I meet a Gurkha, at least I am fairly sure he is a Gurkha – many of these soldiers train in Wales, take a liking to the country and settle here. (A street in Brecon boasting Nepali restaurants is known as Gurkha Tydfil.) He looks me over, searchingly. We exchange nods. I realise he is acting as a bodyguard to someone out of sight, someone I can hear behind a screen.

'Can I . . . see?'

He nods.

I peer around the screen. The man behind it has just struck a drive. He turns and looks at me quizzically. He is a large man with small feet and a pallid brown complexion, a man in late middle age, hefty and unsmiling. I nod. He nods. I apologise for disturbing him and all but tiptoe away.

I am exulted and surging with adrenaline. He was not quite human! His body was too large for his feet. He did not look very well, as well he might not. He is a liaison officer, a go-between. He was either another kind of being, in a form like but unlike us, or he was a human who has spent time negotiating with our extraterrestrial friends. Either way, he seemed like a hostage to the negotiations, someone with a much heavier responsibility than me. Imagine having a Gurkha bodyguard as your minder. The poor man. How fortunate I am to have this wide-ranging role, the freedom.

I feel great relief and renewed pressure. This *is* happening: other people are involved, men and women with families and children – all these people around the world, all of us working, hoping, all relying on each other, and most of us, I assume, isolated, unable to discuss our work or share our burdens. But what a privilege to be allowed to meet that man. I have no doubt that our encounter was intended as a reward and an encouragement. I will do whatever I can, I vow. I will not quit or baulk – I will not give up or be found wanting.

It is dark now. I press north into Snowdonia and the high mountains.

By midnight I am near Machynlleth, the only car on the road. The entire country is deserted. The temperature is well below freezing according to the car, and I am very tired. In a pine forest I find a car park. I think it is some sort of visitor attraction. The temperature in the car will drop rapidly when I turn the engine off. I mummify myself in layers of clothes, heap others over me, wind back the driver's seat and prepare to sleep. Enormous trees crowd around. There is no moon.

The planets are close. In the glittering darkness the stars have a mobile quality, as though the heavens are swinging gently on their hinges.

Four in the morning. The stars have wheeled. Start the engine, boost the heaters, turn and head back to the road. North-west again. I know exactly where I am going – to the end of the land, to the western sea, to the tip of the Llyn Peninsula.

An hour or so later we roll quietly, the car and I, down to the end of a no-through road. A prophet's moon is lifting out of the sea, a swooping crescent glowing gold. It looks like the beginning of the world, this moonrise over an abandoned planet. I watch, becalmed.

Now I turn again and feel my way through the lanes, following the curve of the Llyn to Aberdaron and the end of the land. This is one of my favourite places in all the world. The first time I came here, to the parish where R. S. Thomas lived and wrote, I felt I had come home. Out past Aberdaron, beyond the end of the headland, Ynys Enlli, Bardsey, the island of twenty thousand saints, lies still and miraculous, a place of pilgrimage where the veils between dimensions of belief and perception are thin and all luminous now, under a dawn-blue sky.

A sensible metaphor for breakdown is the lost thread, the broken narrative of being. In a storm of fantasies, fears and paranoias, the beliefs which held you steady have capsized, leaving you in the welter of the present, your course and bearings chaotically scrambled.

Healing, in this view, is the process of restoring that story to you, of putting back together the links of memories and values that form the chain of a life, of righting you like a boat. I suspect the planks of my memories and values had become warped and lost their integrity, so that leaks of guilt, despair, self-loathing and revulsion at my created world sprang between them. Rather than go down with the knackered raft of myself, some part of me seems to have preferred to hurl it all in the air and dive into the chaos beneath.

But the man who now leaves the car and strides down over the headlands towards the sea is easy in the present. I am secure in my memories of coming here, with friends and with pupils from a writing course I brought here once. I have known and loved the Welsh coast since I was a small boy. I have made dawn walks like this, into the simple wonder of the early light, the sea and the birds, every year of my life. The choughs feeding on the clifftop turf are my favourite birds, my totems. The black-backed gulls, the ravens and the rock doves, the gannets out at sea, the kestrels hanging in the winds of the morning are known to me, iterations of life and being I hold sacred.

Fantasies about aliens, world governments, Kylie Minogue, surveillance and secret purposes are nothing to me now. I am experiencing this place, this morning of bright moments, the clifftop rocks and heathers, the smell of the turf and the sea, exactly as they are. I am drinking fresh water where it bubbles up through the rocks on the edge of the sea, the pilgrims' well. I am walking the contour paths of the cliff, looking north-west for a glimpse of the Mountains of Mourne in Ireland, which you can see from here when the conditions are right.

This present elides with my past. If you had met me at that moment, and talked to me, you would have found me calm and secure. As mania shades into psychosis the intensity of the present erases the claims of the past and the calls of the future. I live so vividly in the present that implications and consequences have no hold on me. My sense of self is no longer built like a storyboard, with each frame followed by another, related frame. Instead, the stories of all the versions of me that my imagination can conjure are splashed across packs of different cards, Tarot, Rumi, Monopoly and playing cards all mixed. A short sleep shuffles the cards one way; an insignificant event (in reality) shuffles them another way. Profligate spending and sexual promiscuity make perfect sense – tomorrow is such an infinity of moments and possibilities away that it becomes abstract. Tomorrow could be anything: it could be the Second Coming of Jesus, it could be the end of the world; it may be out there somewhere – who knows?

As the mania intensifies these shuffles from one story to another take place more rapidly. In order to hold myself in some kind of steadiness I cling to the strongest – and, though this seems strange – perhaps the most sensible guiding narrative. (The Security Service exists to watch people; over half the world's population believes in intelligent extraterrestrial life; the US Air Force has released videos of apparent encounters with UFOs; no one has explained what was actually going on with the Gatwick drones – and Kylie is unmarried.)

This may explain why so many of us who have experienced delusions default to similar fantasies. Only in moments like this clifftop morning am I able to release all these improvised, first aid fantasies. The strength of my associations with this place and the brightness of its being return me, for a few hours, to the deeper story of who I am.

On the top of the headland is Mynydd Mawr coastguard lookout, a white hut above a giant and glinting sea. During the war seventy RAF personnel were involved in keeping watch here, tracking shipping and aircraft. There is a photograph of one of the men who worked at the lookout on a plaque on the wall of the hut. He is in uniform, holding a pen over a notepad. He is in his sixties, busy and committed, glancing at the photographer, his mouth caught in terse speech. When you've finished messing with that thing you might like to do some work, he seems to say. I salute him.

The work, the work of watching, waiting, fighting, helping: that is what we must do. The morning is drawing on.

Reluctantly I know I must get back to it, back to work. I take the lanes and roads to the north coast, making for Ynys Mon, Anglesey, the ancient home and last refuge of the Druids. I do not know why I must go there. On the way I stop at a slate museum, slightly alarming the owners by drifting around, ordering breakfast, leaving the table to scout about, coming back, being unable to settle, not having much money.

Back in the car I listen to Georges Brassens, reassured by his gravelly French. Around midday I cross the bridge over the Menai Straits. I have not been to Anglesey since I was a child. It is beguiling, somehow conspiratorial. Its island-in-time feeling and its deep Welshness are spliced with something else: it feels as though there is a resilience here, a resistance to time and the rest of the world. I feel tremendously at home and excited, discovering a new country which abutted mine unsuspected, as if I have stepped through a time shift. I celebrate with a half-pint at the Bulkeley Arms and note the clock stands at quarter to one. From now on, I decide, this will be my benchmark, a firm line drawn in Anglesey: no drinking before quarter to one.

I range down to the shore, slipping and jumping between green weed and rocks, rejoicing in the sweet reek of the mud and vegetation at low tide. I am hungry. The gulls here are enormous. They must do well on the foreshore. Inspired by them I eat seaweed and pick more for the journey. I can feel the surge of goodness and strength as I swallow it. Why am I here? I think of royal weddings and investitures in my childhood. Perhaps that is it: they want to run a christening here, some secret ceremony connected with the ancient claims of the Crown and the counter-claims of the Welsh. I should survey it for them.

At the age of nine and ten I did this sort of thing all the time. I was forever coming up with stories, assigning myself exciting roles and living them in my head, under the unsuspecting gaze of my parents. When I was fourteen or so I was an inspector of nuclear submarine bases. My job was to break into them to test their security. And here I am again, in my mid-forties, a trusted and expert scout for the secret state, half playing and half not playing at surveying the strengths and vulnerabilities of the little town of Menai Bridge, which has been selected to host a covert, or at least very discreet, royal occasion.

The survey takes only as long as you would need to walk a swift circuit of the town and prowl slitheringly along the foreshore, grazing on more seaweed. At last, tired and satisfied with a good day's work, I return to the car and set off for the North, for home, for my poor family.

CHAPTER 7

First contact: police

Our little house sits in the middle of the terrace at the end of the valley, one of the last before the woods. It overlooks a meadow where the beck runs along the base of the Buttress, a swelling lump of hill thickly covered with trees. Small and cramped for four of us, and the dog, it is a lovely place to live, the windows filled with the colours of leaves and weather. The skies and their moods are ever-present.

It is dark when I arrive, hauling the carpet into the front room. Our little boy is asleep in bed. Rebecca and her mother are downstairs. I want to see our child but they do not want me to go upstairs. I retreat back to the flat in town.

The flat has one bedroom but I do not use it. Nightly I make my nest downstairs. It was the same in Wales: I slept in the living room, rather than my bedroom. Everything is in flux. I cannot settle in a bed as though nothing were out of place.

Over the next few days I fix a new geography of Hebden Bridge. Across the road below the flat is Nutclough Mill, now office spaces. Here GCHQ have their headquarters. People between the ages of eighteen and twenty-five are working for them. Everything I say or do in the flat can be monitored from Nutclough. There is a camera in the black radiator on wheels which I move around the living room. There is another in the front of the hi-fi. Others work when the lights are switched on. There is one in the oven. One street behind me is Zaff's house, a safe place. One street behind him is Doug's house.

Hebden is famous for its under-dwellings: the steep gradients up which the houses are built mean west-facing ground-floor flats on one street are effectively the basements of east-facing houses built over them, which open to streets above. Now they are also linked by a system of tunnels. My guess is that many of these houses are connected with passages defended by false walls and secret doors. One of them comes out in the portioned-off space under the stairs in the flat.

In the bedroom and bathroom upstairs you can hear the footsteps of the woman who lives above and the click-click of her dog's nails on her wooden floors. Hers is a safe house occupied by the security services.

There is a strange electronic beep, which sounds every now and then, like a smoke detector running out of battery. The odd thing is there is no smoke detector. I cannot work out where it is coming from or why. It means something, I am sure. I will figure it out.

The whole complex operation in Hebden is being controlled from two large houses up the hill to the north, to the right of the flat. I can see them from my windows. You can be sure they can see me.

I go to see my therapist the day after returning to Yorkshire. It is a long-standing appointment. We have been meeting on and off for a while. For years I feared therapy. The last thing I wanted to do was look at the mess I believed myself to be. Press on, be kinder, work harder, do better: I had a mantra. It was just a question of sticking to it, I hoped. By the winter of 2017 the mantra was in bits. I was depressed and depressing. I sought help. Some of the tools my therapist gave me have helped carry me this far. She has taught me about taking too much responsibility and about neglecting self-care. And she has talked about the window of functionality that exists between threat and panic above (when the frontal cortex cuts out and you cannot make decisions) and catatonia below (where you can do nothing). To remain within this window I need to work from a wellspring of feeling more than thinking, and food, sleep, balance and ease. She has tried to teach me about being good enough, rather than seeking perfection, about releasing stress, about a sense of proportion.

We have worked on childhood trauma, on a period during my parents' divorce and a move to a hill farm with my mother, when I seem to have had hidden feelings of threat and loss and need, concealing them under an appearance of rational understanding. My therapist does not believe that words like bipolar are useful; she believes in exorcising trauma through recovered feeling in order to heal splits in the psyche. She is trying to help me pull up the floors under which I have buried my worthlessness and guilt, to liberate emotion from the grip of thought. She sees mania as an explosion of suppressed feeling, and depression as its price.

We have struggled to make progress. I have found it extraordinarily difficult not to defend my parents, not to justify and rationalise their actions, not to keep the pain and responsibility close to me rather than handing it to my father and mother, as my therapist believes I should.

For a time we stalled. In the last few weeks the greatest value of our sessions has seemed to be that every time I have to tell someone I am OK, saying 'I see a therapist' mollifies them. But I am determined to keep seeing her. I believe in her and what she can do and help me do. We have dates marked down for weeks hence and I am not going to miss one – not one.

Her little room with its scented candles, low light and box of tissues by the client's chair should feel safe. I have just had a joint. I am scared, deep down, that I may not be able to maintain my fiction of well-being. She tells me I am high,

in the manic sense. I do not tell her I am high in the mari-
juana sense. She says she thinks we have come as far as we
can. I need to see a psychiatrist, she says.

'Is this how a therapist dumps a client?' I ask, laughing.

'Well yes,' she says. 'You could say that.'

She wishes me good luck repeatedly, with evident feeling.
So much for therapy, I think.

At night I range the backs and side streets of Hebden,
calling into bars, emptying my pockets, drinking. Late, under
a starry sky, I come across a pile of marble offcuts. Someone
is redecorating a bathroom. Delighted, I scoop up an armful
of marble shards. *Heavy*, I think, *good*. Left out for me on
purpose. Training . . . I jog home with my trophies.

Her face taut with desperation, Rebecca drives us into
town, where I try to sell the rug. The Afghan Rug Shop will
not take it. We go to Todmorden. A corner shop there sells
antiques, bric-a-brac and rugs. The owner is away. The
person minding the shop does not have the authority to buy
it. I can see what is going on here. The smart woman in the
long coat on the other side of the street represents the British
government. By the window the limping Asian boy with his
companion, possibly his carer, is probably Pakistani, working
for the ISI, representing Afghan interests. The big man by
the till looks like a retired naval officer.

'Right,' I announce, 'I'm going to auction this thing now.
Any opening bids? OK, five hundred pounds.'

The naval man looks at me.

'A thousand pounds,' I say, nodding at him.

The woman across the street gesticulates.

'Five thousand pounds.'

The Asian boy dips his head and says something to his
companion. I take it as a bid.

'Ten thousand.'

The naval man looks outraged or bewildered. A police
helicopter goes over, low. It's all happening.

The Asian boy dips his head. We need to finish this. The auction is symbolic. We all know it. The point is to fix a figure – some huge pile of reparation, compensation, treasure, some redress to the maimed and bereft of Afghanistan.

'Fifteen billion pounds, and sold!' I cry, striding dramatically out of the shop.

Clattering and roaring, the helicopter circles low, round and round. There must be many dignitaries and military types in town for this but, even so, the security is intrusive. They must feel they have no choice. Thank God my part is done. They can argue all they like. They have a figure. Let them get on with it. I walk up past the church, round the back of the town, along the lane.

Outside the shop the owner says to Rebecca, 'He's not well, is he?'

'No, he's really not.'

'He needs help, doesn't he?'

'I am trying but he just talks his way out of it.'

'And they let him go? Is it because he's got a posh voice?'

'Yes. And because he knows what to say.'

'You've got no chance,' the man says. 'They hear his voice and they just think, *Oh, he's some kind of eccentric.*'

It is hard to see where the intervention could have come from. If you can make a persuasive or at least coherent case that you are well, it is easy to slip between the different services. The doctor in Brecon was easily evaded: I appeared to have capacity, as the jargon goes. I said I was under the care of a crisis team in the North. It was the festive season – who knows what other pressures he faced?

I found the crisis team very easy to deal with. You told them you were reducing your drug and alcohol intake, you told them you felt fine, you told them you were sleeping well, and on you went. As long as you say you do not think you have special powers, do not hear voices, do not have thoughts of killing yourself, and as long as you present no apparent danger to yourself or others, you are free to roam.

The police helicopter departs. I figure the negotiations will go on but that the most high-value officials and the greatest risks among the delegates have left too. The helicopter's presence joins my bank of evidence. Back into Todmorden I go. Rebecca and I load the rug into the car. Her face is pain brought to a matter-of-factness. 'You're not well,' she keeps saying. 'You're manic, you need help.'

'I'm fine,' I insist. 'Leave me alone.'

Now I am very busy. There is all the news to keep up with, there is an event in London to prepare for – I am due to give a talk about Bach – and the developing situation in Hebden Bridge with which I must keep abreast. Under it all are thoughts of family, which flood me sometimes and which sometimes I push away.

'It will all be worth it,' I keep telling myself. 'The world *will* be a better place for this. One day I will explain it all to my darling boy. This is all for him.'

I speak aloud to myself and my hidden listeners a lot, these days.

I now know that birds can understand me and convey messages, passed from bird to bird, across huge distances. They can communicate progress and developments across the country, across the Channel, across Europe, all the way to the mountains of Pakistan and Afghanistan.

Obsessed with messaging and communication, I hook up an old laptop to the hi-fi in the flat, and connect that to a radiator by means of wires. Now I can receive messages via Radio 4 and the Internet and transmit by talking to the microphones and cameras which survey and record everything I do in the flat.

My sanctuary is a slit of space behind the bathroom, just wide enough for a desk. I have decorated it with maps, postcards, business cards, bottle tops, enamel bird badges, more maps.

The bathroom I believe to be off camera but on microphone. I spend a lot of time in here, showering in the dark or bathing in candlelight. At one point I waterboard myself using a wet facecloth over which I pour glasses of water, just to see what it is like. It is a strange and urgent time. When night falls the mania rises like a tide. The delusions become narrower and more powerful.

Six o'clock, the news. I must listen and comment. Quarter past seven, *Front Row*, for which I used to work. (It is particularly easy to convince yourself that the radio is talking to you when the presenters are friends and adept at broadcasting as though they *are* talking to you.) Then out and ranging around until *The World Tonight* at ten, and not forgetting the midnight news.

Every time the transmissions come from Parliament, which is locked in furious debate over Brexit, I must be on duty. John Bercow, Ken Clarke and Yvette Cooper are my allies. My enemies are theirs. I develop a habit of smoking strong joints (strong by my standards) when listening to Parliament, in the belief that they help facilitate different kinds of perception and communication. Some sort of universal consciousness is arising, I can feel it, I am certain of it, and my brain is a node in this vast and majestic new system which is taking human communication and compassion to a new dimension.

As I become stoned in my flat, parliamentarians in Westminster feel the same things I do, their thoughts slowing and brightening, their sympathy widening, their senses of humour broadening. The presenter Neil Nunez has a gorgeous voice. When he is reading the continuity links, I can feel my stoned brain meshing with his, both of us smiling and drifting, euphoric. Ken Clarke and John Bercow often seem as high as me, making the House laugh or roar in outrage, sometimes intervening, it seems, randomly.

My understanding of Rebecca's position flowers. I see how hard she is trying – I just have not been able to understand her place in everything. Now I know that she is part of this too. I believe that her moral clarity and her perspective are vital to the great undertaking. I admire her absolutely, her knowledge (she reads far more than I do), her angles on politics, gender and society. I understand that balance and integrity mean that we cannot be together – she has to make her own judgements on the news and the crisis in Parliament, and they will be recorded (of course our house is bugged) and balanced with my take. This, I realise, is why she locks the door when I appear in the lane. She needs to hear the radio news uninfluenced by me.

As I range over the hills and around the town at night, on my fierce training programme, Rebecca, who is an ultra-runner, is following her own regime, running and strengthening. Like me, she comes from a family which is part of the secret state.

'I know who you are working for,' I tell her mother. 'I've given you your card. You are out.'

I believe that Rebecca's parents, who are a dear and widely beloved couple, have been senior figures in the MI5 operation in Rochdale for many years.

'I know what she was doing in Portugal,' I tell her mother. 'When I first met her, she was scared of knives. I knew she was working with gangsters. Now I know she was reporting on them too, and I think they caught her, and I think she had to be rescued, and I believe she has post-traumatic stress, and I think it's rotten they haven't looked after her properly.'

The thought of what they have done to her makes me cry with rage. Rebecca and her mother are speechless. I make another exit.

I keep trying to see my little boy. One night I manage to get as far as the bedroom in our house. There he is, my

beautiful little son, five years old, in his pyjamas, sitting on
the double bed where he sleeps with his mother, guarded
now by his grandmother, his hair tousled, the room a wreck
(Rebecca is reorganising the house in my absence). He looks
like a small angel of light and he hugs me.

'I love you so much, darling,' I tell him.

'I love you too, Dad,' he says, and we squeeze each other
tight.

'It will all be over soon,' I say, 'It will all be all right.'

'You've got to go, Dad,' he says.

'I know, darling. I love you.'

I go up to the attic. I make a pile of all his older brother's
stuff, hundreds of pounds' worth of speakers and headphones
and leads and phones and tablets. The poor boy has been
engulfed by GCHQ, deluged with all this bugged and
betraying equipment.

'It's moody,' I tell the teenager, such a gentle, beloved
soul, who now looks driven to desperate anguish by his work
for the security services. 'Get rid of it all.'

He is aghast, enraged and distressed by what I am doing
to his mother, by the pain, the conflict and the betrayals I
have wrought.

His father in Rochdale comes on the phone.

'Get out of the house,' he tells me. 'Horatio, get out of
the house.'

I hang up on him. I start moving things around in the
attic, turning the mattress over, clearing a space and inad-
vertently, carelessly trashing the room. I lie down on the
mattress for a few moments, my eyes closed.

Rebecca calls the police.

Three officers find me in the front room. Their uniforms
and the equipment on their belts are intimidating: the house
feels as though it might burst. But they are level-headed.
They establish that Rebecca does not want me in the house,
and that there is somewhere else I could go.

'Let's calm this whole situation down,' says the woman police officer. She stays with Rebecca while two young male constables drive me down to town. They are friendly, easy, laid-back. As I will discover, a huge proportion of their time is spent dealing with people in mental distress.

'Do you get any help – I mean counselling?' I ask one of the officers as he escorts me from the patrol car to the door of the flat. 'Your job must be very traumatic sometimes.'

'It can be,' he says. 'Yeah, it is.' Something seems to be tearing behind his eyes. I can only imagine what he has seen and had to do, but I can clearly see the effect on him. There is hell and distress behind his gaze.

This is something else about madness: there is no hiding from it. 'Look in my eyes and lie to me,' becomes one of my catchphrases around now. Nobody does.

The police officers of Halifax and the Calder Valley are some of the heroes of this story. In what is coming, they will repeatedly put themselves out, go that little bit further, stay beyond their shifts. They do everything they possibly can to support Rebecca and to protect her and me from me.

CHAPTER 8

Night walking

I am now escalating. On a street I find a packet of prescription medication, blue pills in a blister pack. I assume it is Ecstasy – evidently they want to trial the Dutch model on me, whereby pills are tested for purity. I am to be the guinea pig. Fair enough. I can take it. (When Rebecca discovers the packet she looks up the name of the medication – it is for herpes.) In the meantime it is crucial to get the peace and cooperation treaties signed. I believe the conflict between Rebecca and me is a microcosmic version of the conflict between nations. I go to see my solicitor.

'I want to go for custody of my son,' I say. 'Rebecca will go for full custody. If I don't do anything I won't be able to see him. So I'll go for full and hopefully we will get joint.'

My solicitor is a wise and careful person. She specialised in divorce when she was in London, before moving to Hebden and, she says, a better life. She would be a brilliant divorce and separation advocate; I can see her looking for the best and kindest solution for the whole family – for us. We had a fascinating conversation when I was sane, about how a divorce solicitor would handle Brexit. Now, clearly, she is engaged in the secret negotiations at the highest level.

'I really wouldn't go down this route,' she says. 'You can never tell what is going to happen – courts make mistakes. They make bad judgements. I would absolutely urge you to go through mediation, to work it out between yourselves. It is honestly, honestly the best course.'

Paperwork is key, I realise. We must get everything right. My son's school has put out a call for parents who are interested in standing for election to the board of governors. I post a ballot paper to the headmistress with an extra box drawn on it, Rebecca's name added to it, and the box ticked. (The headmistress will never mention it.)

The following few days seem now like a chaotic, cyclonic poem, the memories dreamlike and unnaturally bright. What did I do? In the Robin Hood, which was jammed with revellers, I gave minute signals of assent to secret, violent missions by the special forces. I knew the moral responsibility was on me. Outside the Packhorse Inn on the moors I met a man who worked with the Irish coastguard – he told me of men lost in storms against the cliffs, and I believed he was telling me of the cost in lives of missions I had sanctioned, and I agonised. I took the 'Ecstasy' I had found in the street. I ran into my friend Ben Myers. We went for coffee and suddenly the 'Ecstasy' hit. I could hear the thoughts of everyone in the café. Ben, assuming I was on something, was a rock. We talked about writing. He lent me money. I think I would have collapsed in the café had it not been for the steadiness of his sympathy, a feeling that he knew exactly where I was. For a short while I felt I had nothing to hide. The rush of that all but took my legs away.

I communed with former lovers psychically in my flat. I began to hack a hole in the back of the cupboard under the stairs with a knife because it was a trapdoor to a secret passage where one of them was hiding.

I had sex with shadow versions of this memory or that memory in the shower, in candlelight, and I felt humiliated because I believed I was being watched.

In a café I believed the women of the town were telling me that a popular and respected figure was a criminal dangerous to children, and I gave my assent for his murder, an extrajudicial killing carried out by the state on my authority. I wept and tore scabs off my legs and toes in penance.

There was a system now, a sin-eating system, in which terrible things would be confided to me, communicated with a combination of subtle signs and inferences, and I would sanction redress and punishment and murder, and bleed and suffer for my presumption.

Around this time I took the discarded Christmas tree from outside the house of friends and put it outside Zaff's flat. Later I erected it sloppily outside mine. I left a bag of clothes outside Zaff's door, and wine. I spent some quiet time with him during which I almost passed as sane, apart from feeling I must throw certain of his Rumi cards into his fire.

I engaged in races around the town, trying to make peace and bridge conflicts. In the Tibetan restaurant I prayed for justice for Tibet and redress from China. I bought a beautiful edition of Shakespeare's collected works and left it in the lavatories of the Old Gate pub. I signed a box of copies of my book on Bach and believed they would be extraordinarily valuable, a common codebook for all the forces and services, the soldiers, spies and negotiators who swirled around me. I put them out on the street near the bus stop where the school children gather, in the hope that they would help themselves. (Gallingly, none did.) I fought sleep and waking, made love to ghosts, believed the footsteps in the flat above belonged to an ex-lover.

In the White Lion I saw a friend from London, a vicar's son (he actually was there). I still believed that a royal christening was taking place in secret in the town and that I must make it safe, and I raced around the valley by night and day, patrolling. I posted insane rantings on Facebook. One night I went up to the moors.

Go into the crisp dark bright of it, into the frost and the sparkle, up the road to the moor. The land below is a black inlet, the moon high and the woods a reef. Mazy coves of trees sway along the contours, the valleys below lost in silvery gloom. Follow the path to a field which mutters with the sound of shifting hooves. Pause here, perch on a gate, guess, go diagonally, and now into another field with more animals in it – are they goats? Black goats or black sheep. A scurry of them. Go quietly. Hello, goats! They act strangely. Not frightened of me but dithery and curious. Odd. Another wall beyond them – different this one, the heavy stones not pains-takingly fitted but more a crumbly stack of them. Go over slowly, carefully, into a wood's edge, small rowans, tight here, ungrazed, fairy territory, moss and a different darkness. And then . . . stop. The ground sloping to nothing. Pine tops coming up from below. Hard to see but there is . . . Yes! There is nothing at all. I am on the lip. Move slowly, hold the twigs, crane and peer. Fifty feet fall. Hard to turn with the roots and boles there. No way forward, no way sideways. Stay still. Inch. Keep low. Slither back to the crumbly wall. Follow it very carefully. Hello, goats! Yes, I see. I do see now. Thank you for the warning. Thank you.

And now the reward, springing moss and birches, a path only foxes know, and the descent and below that the road back to town, exhilarated.

For a long moment I thought about climbing down the cliff. I would have fallen. So there is still a switch there, below all the tangled wiring. It still works. Go. Don't go. Don't live. Live.

And I meet Richard. He comes along the road through the wood as the light is fading. Tall and handsome, his clothes loose, he has a limber quietness. I have seen him before around the town but we have never spoken. I am perching on the wall. I have been crying and cursing.

'There you are!' I say. 'Hello.'

'Hello,' he says, smiling as if not quite taken by surprise. His voice is soft and burred like moss on stone. I tell him my name and guess his, which makes him laugh.

'I'm sorry,' I say. 'I'm in a bit of a state. I was just thinking about my sister. She died in 2011. I was just thinking about her and Seamus Heaney, "From the Republic of Conscience".'

He listens. When I finish he waits a while and says gently, 'You're in grief.'

'It's true. I think I am. I told myself that grief lasts two years and that I was out of it. How do you get through?'

He answers nothing quickly.

'I walk. I keep on a level. I don't see too many people. I keep silence.'

'What can I do?'

'Listen to what's in here,' he says, touching his chest. 'Take some time. Don't do anything you don't want to do.'

'It's taken me such a long time to be here,' I say. 'I feel guilty about being here, about writing here, because it's not my place.'

'You're very welcome, Horatio,' he says, soft.

'I've never dared write poetry here!'

'You are a poet,' he says. 'Walk. Look.' He gestures to the trees. 'Be with this. You'll be all right.'

'Where are you going?'

'You can't come where I'm going,' he says, laughing. 'I'm going to a teepee, actually.'

'Of course you are!'

We laugh and hug.

His hand seems to leave a warm imprint between my shoulders. It is the strangest thing, mighty and gentle, a touch that seems to come through time somehow, like a passing-on. He walks away and I go down to the beck in the dark.

Keep silent, I tell myself, keep silent and listen. You are a poet. Be with the beck and the stars, the trees and the dark. Don't do anything you don't want to do. Keep silent and listen to the trees. It will be all right. Listen to what is in here.

The beck runs glittering black under an overhang, under threatening, teetering masses of rock and stark trees outlined against the night. The cold is bright and vivifying. I perch on a rock and believe in good energy, in transfer through time, in poetry.

Through what was to come I tried to remember what he said. I tried to follow his advice. I recalled the feel of the touch between my shoulders. I tried to keep silence, to hold to a stillness in my core. Poet! That night it was licence, reprieve, release. Poets are allowed to walk the woods at night, to commune with the dead. You will be OK. Walk. Be with this. You will be all right.

Richard listened without judgement. Nothing I said seemed to alarm him. His manner and voice were soothing. He engaged with me as though I was as valid as he was, as ill or un-ill as he was. His advice was sensible and helpful: look for stillness, give silence time, do not be frightened, be hopeful, believe that all in the end will be well. I could not have had more than ten minutes of his wisdom. I needed years.

CHAPTER 9

Crash

Now it feels as though I am telling the story of the last days of my life. From the slit-room with the maps behind the bathroom I can send messages around the world. See – I tap on the south-facing wall and a few moments later there is a tick from the north wall behind me. I do it again on the east wall; now comes a noise from the west.

Soon it will be time to collect our rewards for all the exhausting work we have done. I walk around Hebden selecting a car for Robin, who is old enough to take his driving test. An Audi, I decide. He is a wonderful boy who has been through a lot, an awful lot.

The prize for his mother and me will be one of our dreams made true. We have long talked, idly, about starting a school. Rebecca is an extraordinary teacher, qualified to director of studies level. The United World College of the Pennines will fill all these flats and buildings, linked by stairs and cut-throughs which are just waiting to be exposed. I begin work on the tunnel under the stairs, cutting through the plasterboard with a kitchen knife. We are hours away from the last great conference of the secret negotiations. My father and his partner will be coming to stay in the White Lion. I think they may already be here. We will all process through one another's houses, dancing and celebrating. I clear my front room and kitchen, making space for the great party. Everyone I love will be coming.

A piece of paper arrives from my bank. I have lost track of my spending but it looks as though the Security Service is taking care of business for me. On the letter there are three rejected payments, one of which is the mortgage. Beside each is written, 'Refer to Debtor,' but I read them as 'Refer to Director.' I am lightly dyslexic and much distracted, so I give it no more than a glance, just enough time to misread it. I am reassured by the director's intervention. You see? It is all true.

Strange noises at night. People moving in the secret passages behind the walls and overheard. They are clearing out the safe houses and listening posts all around, leaving just a skeleton crew to take care of security for the final conference. Very soon now I will be quite alone, all these flats deserted except for a few watchers and soldiers.

Up to our family house in the woods I go. Our neighbour, Liz, lets me into her house. I am swigging from a champagne bottle. She finds me frightening. When I try to get into our house Rebecca calls the police again. How easy it was to be the cause of so much trouble, and what hell it was to be subjected to it. A year later, almost to the night, Rebecca recalls it.

'That was the night you were at Ellie and Doug's, dressed really weirdly. You had been talking about your sister and when you left you said, "Give my love to my son." So they thought you were going to kill yourself. That was the night Bushra and Sue came over from Rochdale looking for you. That was the night Scott and Stuart and Alistair were all out looking for you. The boys from the White Lion were out looking for you. Gary was out looking for you. People went round all the pubs in Hebden looking for you. And all the time you were at Liz's drinking champagne and whisky and God knows what and making comments about how you'd like to shag people on TV. [Liz's house is a few doors down from ours.] Liz was really scared. Then you knocked

on the door and said you were the police and I let you in.
You went upstairs and you were saying you were going to
take your child. Then you had a bath, and me and Liz were
blocking the door to the bedroom and my mum was in the
bedroom blocking the door from the inside. And you threw
my Buddha into the field and you left and the police picked
you up in the wood. We were calling the crisis team and
they were useless. When the policeman was here he spoke
to them and they said, "If he's just drunk there's nothing
we can do." I said of course he smells of alcohol, he poured
champagne all over my keyboard. The policeman told them,
"He's just poured alcohol over his partner's keyboard but
quite how much he's drunk we're not willing to say. It seems
performative." He was funny, actually, the policeman.
Bushra and Sue were here and he said, "I'm getting all these
big words tonight from you lot." He said, "I'll take down
everything you've all said and hopefully the psychiatrist
won't discharge him."

'They took you to Halifax and you were interviewed by a
psychiatrist who let you go. The poor policeman was
wonderful. When he finished his shift he came round. It was
about five in the morning and he'd said he'd ring me. He
knocked on the door and he said. "I am so sorry, I am so
sorry but they've let him go. He's talked his way out of it
again." He said, "I've told him, if you go round there again
it doesn't matter if your partner's saying it's mental health,
we'll charge you with domestic abuse." He was really lovely.
He gave me the number of a friend of his who's a solicitor
in Halifax and said, "I really think you need to take out a
restraining order."'

Rebecca and I have talked all this through and through.
When I first heard the words 'domestic abuse' I was appalled.
I do not believe myself even remotely capable of abuse. They
did not think I meant to do them harm but they feared that
in my madness I might harm all or any of us – I had no

intention of taking my son from the house that night, in my memory. I wanted to see him, I wanted to fight for custody of him in the future, but I do not believe I wanted physical possession of him or to be responsible for him that night or at any moment in that horrendous time. I was far too selfish for that, and too committed to the idea of doing something which would allow me to return to him as the hero I longed to be. Rebecca did not see what was happening as abuse, which is a comfort, but then many abused women do not see their abusers in these terms. The police are probably the best judges of such a situation: in their experience I am at this point one visit short of the line.

Rebecca says, 'You *did* want to take him, you did keep coming round, you wanted to be in the house. You did say you wanted to take him, which was why my mum was sitting on a laundry basket behind the door. Robin was formidable on every occasion, and so kind to you.'

I remember the drive to Halifax in the police van. I remember waiting to be seen by someone and I remember being driven back. I have no memory of telling whoever interviewed me that I was fine, only of being believed. I remember being driven back to the flat.

Tonight it is all happening: the radio has tipped me off. On *Front Row*, John Wilson is talking to Charlie Brooker about *Bandersnatch*, the latter's interactive dystopian TV series, and reviewing the shortlist for the Costa Awards.

By talking to the radio I believe I have negotiated a win for Zaffar Kunial for his luminous poetry collection *Us*. Rebecca will be the head of the new college in Hebden. I might get a travel prize for my book on walking in the footsteps of J. S. Bach. All will be well, all will be so very well. I tune out when Sophie Raworth on *Front Row* announces that the poetry prize has gone to another writer. I am not really able to process or even really hear information which does not concur with my delusions.

Bandersnatch, John Wilson says, tells the story of a computer games programmer who creates an interactive game. Viewers of the programme make choices on behalf of the protagonist as they watch.

'How many different permutations of the story are there?' Wilson asks.

'I don't know,' Brooker replies.

'Netflix claims a trillion,' Wilson observes.

'That strikes me as . . . optimistic,' says Brooker.

They are talking about us, about this, about me. The programme is being broadcast live from somewhere close by – possibly in the Nutclough studios over the road. Brooker and Wilson are talking about *this* great enterprise, about the relationship between the protagonists and the various agencies from different countries who have been involved with us.

'It got so bewilderingly complex there were bits of it we still don't know how to access,' Brooker tells us. That will be the chaotic element – my secret, unobserved exploits.

'A character becoming aware of the fact choices are being made for them . . .' he explains.

Oh yes. It is wonderful, this. I feel as though the whole thing has been explained to me on a technical level. Hugely reassured, energised and full of direction and certainty, I switch the radio off. There it is – that is how they are doing it. Various actors and protagonists playing different parts, acting and interacting with me according to mysterious rules.

Up, out and at 'em! But first I must do my bit for the party, for the great communal meal. I fill a roasting dish with vegetables, spices and seasoning and set it to cook. Then down in the town I am stalking and spying, flitting from the shadows to the light-pooled stairways which remind me of Paris. It's tonight! It's all happening tonight – I can feel it!

My brother, his son and ex-wife will be coming in from America. My aunt and cousins will arrive with my mum. My friends from the BBC will already be here. My writing friends will be incoming – this is a huge, *Bandersnatch*-style game of hide and seek, characters all brought together in one place and then set free to roam, a kind of game of tag, in which we will all end up dancing until dawn in the Trades Club.

I think I spy my friend Robert passing in a small car. I am quite sure my friend Robin has arrived on his narrowboat. In the park I catch sight of Vladimir Putin leaving, stalking away in his long black coat like the Devil, a shadow figure between the street lights. The deal must have been done. I had better run one more check. I jump on a train to Mytholmroyd. I am sure my brother's American ex-wife is on it, and her family. We are not allowed to just walk up to each other – for security we must appear to run into each other.

At Mytholmroyd I leave the train and double back, moving along the railway line, checking the bridges for bombs and sabotage. All well, all safe. On the outskirts of Hebden, at a distance, I see Judi Dench and Theresa May walking arm in arm. It's really happening!

These are not quite hallucinations – they are glimpsed far enough away for certain identification to be impossible. So in outline I see my aunt and cousin Hughie, also walking arm in arm. I feel joyful relief that it is all over and we can all sit down and share our stories and dance until dawn and be happy evermore.

No one comes to my house, at which I am a little surprised. I have it all laid out, veg roasted, rooms cleared, music playing. Never mind. They must want me to go to them first. I switch off the oven, hardly glancing at the camera I know watches me from under its glass hood, and set off down to the Trades Club.

The Trades' atmosphere is distinctive – accepting and loquacious, it is the sort of place which demands you speak up for yourself when called upon. Thankfully the exhaustion is catching up with me and I can manage little more than a couple of drinks and polite nods. I am so moved by what I find here: not my friends and family but another family, consisting of secret friends, my watchers, the incognito legion who have followed me, observed me and taken care of me all this time. And here they all are, from eighteen-year-olds to the bright-eyed elderly, with just one huge in-joke between us: the tall young man in the GCHQ T-shirt.

Later, I find myself in the bedroom of the flat, jumping at shadows as flecks of light on the walls and ceiling are used to communicate with me. This is a new kind of game, the next level, not done with sound or speech but with signals of light and impulses in the brain. I am crouching down in the corner of the room. The lights are off, the curtains open. I have been moving as quietly as a ghost-hunter. And now I see it, a shadow play on the wall.

In the milky orange wash of the street lights outside, projected in grey shadows through the dark room onto the white wall of the bedroom, I am shown an animation.

At first it is comic. Using the same iconography as the Red Bull adverts, a saintly figure with wings and a halo flutters from left to right. Then there is the manger, and the wise men, and the nativity scene. Now there are rockets, great ICBMs lifting off, threatening to end the world. Now a great screwdriver descends and turns the planet, adjusting it. A great big wagging finger hangs over the globe – a mighty and terrible warning. The show ends. Now you know. It's either seismic change or the end of all of us. Act.

I take a bite out of a green strip of card. It is probably LSD. Why someone would plant it in a child's Christmas card I cannot tell. How incredibly, stupidly dangerous. It is lucky they left it in the flat, not the house. The radio tells me to leave a candle burning and a cushion near it. I distinctly remember asking aloud if I should burn the flat down and the answer coming back, partly from the radio, partly from my thoughts, no, leave that to the professionals. They will take care of all the bugs and cameras. You get out of the house. Leave the door unlocked.

I plunge down one side of the valley and up the other. My car is parked in Heptonstall, for some reason. It is time I got on the road. I will go to Liverpool first, then on to London, where I am due to give a reading and do an interview.

I am finding new routes, new secret ways through Hebden. Up through gardens and ginnels, over fences and walls, holding to a straight line I climb, half expecting to see my flat explode below me on the other side of the valley. My car seems to be waiting for me, a loyal friend, ready for adventure.

The moors are dark and silent tonight, my headlights waving white arms at the sky. I follow the road's lifts and dips behind Heptonstall, along the brows of the valley, our valley, towards Widdop. In the stone-old quiet, farms roost over their steep fields. The world is deserted, the houses, the roads; even the sky is clear of the lights of planes. Perhaps everyone has been moved out. Perhaps everything has been shut down. I am taking messages from the radio again. Near the reservoir I pull off the road. While they are cleaning my house of microphones and cameras the car is still lousy with them.

I have been subject to too many competing interests, taken too many orders, been manipulated too much. I am done with it all and I have a picture in my mind of the car going fast over a lip of ground.

Fast, fast over the lip of ground, the seat belt undone and the seat set well back, out of range of the airbag. I want to be braced for the splash, not knocked about by the bag.

The windows are open. The car tilts and drops sickeningly into a rush of white and black, light and water and a splash like a giant's punch. The headlights fumble in the depths and the windscreen is liquid green. Rushing icy water floods in like liquid darkness but I am prepared for the shock. I am holding my breath and I have only one thing to do, one thing to accomplish after so much struggle, after so much pain and loneliness. I must get out. Out through the window. Don't fight through the pouring water. Wait a little, wait for the equilibrium, wait for the car to fill as it sinks, don't fight against it, but for God's sake, for your son's sake, don't breathe in. Keep your breath. Keep your strength – and now, now, *go*. Swim for it. *Swim for your life*. Get to the surface and you are free, free of it all. The cold smashes your muscles, paralyses your muscles, but you will not quit. You will not die now. Up to the air and *gasp*.

You've done it. You lived. There's the bank and you can do it. It's so close you want to laugh and shout, you've done it. God but that was *mad*! But you lived, you lived, you lived. You crawl out of the reservoir, racked with shivers, and alive, and free.

I am still sitting in the car in the lay-by a few hundred metres below the dam.

'I want confirmation,' I say to the radio. 'You want me to run this car off the road?'

The programme is a profile of someone whose name I missed but I recognise the voice of the speaker. It is the elderly academic we met when we were skiing, the Liverpudlian talent spotter and agent runner for MI6.

'Oh yes, he was incredibly brave,' he says.

'Right.'

I take my seat belt off, engage first gear and let the clutch up ever so slowly. The car begins to roll. Its course will take it over rough but flat ground to the lip. There is nothing beyond the edge there but a steep drop. The car is moving well now. I open the door and roll out. I stand and watch the tail lights disappear. The noise changes, there are rattles and thumps, fading now, then a resonant crash.

Silence.

I take off my clothes, retaining only my boots. I want to shed, to help them lay their false trail, or whatever it is they want with this faked car accident. It's almost over. I follow the car's track to the lip and down.

Miraculously, the vehicle has come to rest like a bridge across an overflow drain from the dam. The car is just longer than the concrete channel is wide, so it sits resting on its bumpers a few feet above the shallow channel of water in the bottom of the drain. I climb up into the driver's seat. The car is well built, a Toyota, and it seems unharmed. The lights are still on. The engine has cut out. The radio still plays.

'He was a hero,' the voice is saying. 'He really gave it everything. He got a bash in the face, broke his nose, and he just played on.'

Of course. They want me to complete the staging of this accident. Right then. I kick violently against the windscreen above the steering wheel, roughly where my head might have struck had the airbag failed. It takes a lot of kicks to make it star and crack. Now I take one of my son's boxing gloves. To complete the illusion – which must be crucial to the negotiations or they would never ask it so explicitly of me – I must sustain injuries. I punch myself hard in the centre of my face, and again, until I hear my nose click. That's enough. Fuck them if it's not enough. I trudge back up to the road.

There is a moon behind cloud, no stars. Although I am only wearing my boots it is not that cold. Too cold to stand around, though. I start jogging back along the road towards Hebden. Surely they will pick me up soon. They won't want to leave me out here like this, I hope.

Thank goodness! There. A great big white camper van. How kind of them, how clever – the perfect camouflage. The passenger door opens. I climb in. Immediately there are shouts. 'Someone's just got in! Who are you? Get out!'

There are two women inside, and children. I jump out, terrified. 'Get the hell out! Go away!'

Confused and frightened I circle it – surely they are here for me? Isn't it time I met someone behind all this, someone who can tell me my part is over, that I have done well, that I can go home and sleep? Isn't it time someone in authority sat down with Rebecca and me and said it is all over? Haven't we earned the right to have each other back and be with our little boy?

The camper van starts its engine and lurches at me, chasing me out of the way.

Flee. Run the other way this time, towards the reservoir and the moors.

Keep your spirits up. Don't be shaken. Don't be scared. There is a light up ahead, a farm.

The curtains are open. Soft stair light falls into a dim front room. It looks lovely. How to attract attention? Am I supposed to attract attention or am I supposed to let myself in? Difficult, being naked. Easy to give the wrong impression . . .

Around the side of the house there is a yard. Suddenly the night blazes white, security lights flood on with a roar of barking dogs. At least half a dozen dogs are lined up in cages next to a parked Land Rover, going berserk. I am not going to wait for someone to press a button and release them. They will start with the most vulnerable bits. I jump at the

Land Rover and scramble up to its roof. Now lights come on in the house. The door opens and a man comes out.

He is a young man, fit-looking and perhaps slightly military, like a gamekeeper.

'What the fuck are you doing on there?'

'I think I'm in need of assistance.'

'Get off there. Get down.'

I do. 'I just need help,' I say.

He shuts the door. He looked irritated and incredulous. Not in on it, then. I jog off down the road again, heading back towards Hebden once more.

Not long afterwards a police car appears.

Thank God.

At last.

'What's going on?' one of the officers asks. It is a surprising opening. Aren't they supposed to know? If they do not know I should not tell them. I guess all this needs to be deniable. I need a cover story until I can see their senior officers, the Security Service or the special forces – whoever is party to what is really happening. I will know them immediately.

'I'm not really sure. I think someone left some drugs in my flat and I was driving and I think I just came up on acid. I crashed my car.'

'Where's the car?'

'It's over there – it went over the ledge over there.'

'Are you hurt?'

'I had a bang on the head but I'm fine.'

'You better get in.'

The back seat of that police car is the warmest, softest, most lovely place. The officers cast about with their torches.

'Hey, I've found his clothes over here!'

They bring them; jeans, a jumper and shirt, boxers.

'You better put them on. Bet you're glad we found those.'

It was a remark they made more than once. They were good-humoured. I told them I was very grateful.

'There's a vehicle down there!' another officer calls. A second police car turns up.

After various exchanges and a conversation over the radio it is established that I can be taken in. I am told I am being arrested on suspicion of driving under the influence. I nod contentedly. I am blissfully tired and calm. I think I sleep.

CHAPTER 10

Cell

There is a military-looking policeman who seems to be in charge. Around him, behind the front desk in Halifax police station, various officers are milling, typing on computers, looking me over uninterestedly.

Police forces spend an enormous and increasing slice of their budget dealing with the mentally ill. Over the county boundary, in Lancashire, the chief constable put the figure at 20,000 response hours – 29 per cent of his force's total.

The difficulty for the officers this evening is that it is unclear whether I am unwell or on drugs. I stick to my story, which I think I believe. How else to explain it? Our flat had been let out. I took a tab of green paper. While I was driving I came up on acid and crashed the car.

They put me in a cell. My first thought is that I ought to break out of it. In the corner on the floor are the remains of a previous occupant's meal. The cup fits perfectly in the cell's lavatory. I flush it twice and it overflows. I press the call button.

'The cell is flooding,' I report. 'The toilet's blocked.'

Patiently they move me to the cell next door.

There is a high window of opaque and armoured glass. There is a mirrored hemisphere in one corner which I assume contains a camera. There is a sleeping ledge, moulded to the concrete wall, with a thin blue plastic mattress on it. I ask for a duty solicitor and my named contact – Emma, our friend who lives in town.

The night passes in fifteen-minute sleeps. I seem only to be able to sleep for exactly a quarter of an hour at a time. I see three medical professionals. An Asian doctor asks me to balance on one foot and touch my nose with my eyes closed. A Russian doctor (he certainly speaks some Russian, because I greet him in the language and he replies) takes blood samples. A sympathetic white Yorkshire woman wearing an NHS ID card interviews me and takes details.

'You can tell them from me you're fine, in perfect health,' she says.

The Asian doctor seems distressed by me and I tell him, cheerfully, to cheer up.

The Russian doctor discusses various things people take. I assume by now that I have been spiked – that the story I am telling is true. I am wired and jumpy. It is difficult to be still and calm.

'People take all sorts of things – LSD, Ecstasy, spice . . .' he says.

Christ, I think, *the bastards really did me.* At the same time, I am reassured by his presence. If the Russians are here it means that the negotiations are still going on. They are perhaps claiming me for their own, or at least standing guard over me against whatever the Americans are up to. That white camper van was the Americans, for sure.

'I don't get it,' a female custody officer says. 'You're all over the place, but every time I speak to you [I am pressing the call button a lot, determined to get out of the cell] you can tell me the time to the nearest minute.'

'I used to work for the BBC,' I tell her. 'I'm good with time.'

There are strange moments in the police station. There is the officer who takes my fingerprints who rolls and smears my fingers through the ink. I think he is deliberately blurring the prints. I believe the staged accident on the moors and what is happening here are of a piece. The security services are after someone, some desperate and vicious terrorist whose guilt is assured but against whom they have no proof. They need my crashed car, my DNA and these blurred prints to construct a case against him. And then, waiting on a bench in the reception area of the station, I am for a few moments side by side with a young man of my build, a man with dark and desperate eyes, and I think, *Yes, of course, you're in this too*. We're both part of the same story. We are both suffering for our service.

In the cell I do what I can remember of yoga. I do stretches and press-ups. I run on the spot. I try to remember ballet positions. I sing. I curl up under the mattress and sleep for quarter-hours that feel like dark snaps of time. I have no idea what hour of the night Emma and the solicitor turn up. Our exchanges and interviews become confused. I think they want me to say certain things but I am sure I should stick to my story.

'If you just say you're mad, I can get you out of here,' says the solicitor. He is a friendly and charming man whose legs seem weak, too small for his body. He sits down a lot. I suspect he may be an extraterrestrial. I suspect he is as much in custody here as I am.

Finally, in the small hours of the morning, I am discharged into the care of a bushy-haired man with a long coat, which he wears with a big scarf – a bohemian mature student. I assume he is with MI6. He says his name is Philip. Philip is very sympathetic.

'We're going to take you to a place where you can get care and treatment,' he says outside. 'Would you like a cigarette?'

'God, yes please.'

'If you go and stand over there, just there,' says the policeman with him, 'you can have one, then I'll pick you up.'

Philip and the policeman drive around in a van and pick me up, having sweetly waited for me to finish.

'Do we have to go to this place?' I ask when they tell me we are going to drive to Wakefield. 'Can't I go home?'

'We think you need to see a doctor,' says Philip.

'We won't be long,' says the policeman. 'We'll be there soon.'

Our destination is a hospital car park in the dead of night. We cross wet tarmac under floodlights to a glass door and a reception desk behind it. There is some faffing with codes for the car park: you have to take a printed strip of paper with the code on it from a box to allow you to get out. I palm two, just in case. A corridor with wood and pastel colours. A male nurse. An examination in a surgery, complete with an ECG. I make the doctor laugh, if he is a doctor, and the female nurse too, getting the giggles from the tape they stick to me and asking whether they are charging me up or powering me down. They give me a pill of some sort. I take it. They show me to a room. I black out.

It is a grey day and I am in a small room, facing a 'discharge interview'. The interviewer is a large man whose face I later struggle to picture; he seems harassed and uncertain but I am concentrating very hard on getting out of here. This is a psychiatric hospital, with locked wards for men and women and criminals judged to be mentally ill. This section feels innocuous. It is quite new, with pastel plastic, new chairs and a small number of patients, all men, who mill around in the corridors, their skin made sallow by the yellowish overhead light. I run through my symptoms – cyclothymia, stress, relationship breakdown, seasonal affective disorder – and my remedies.

'I take vitamin D and omega threes. I have reduced my drug and alcohol intake. Last night I took something; I didn't know what it was, I didn't even know if it was a drug or not. People I don't know have been staying in the flat where I live – I thought they might have left drugs there. I was driving over the moors when it hit me, and I think it was strong acid. The next thing I know I've crashed my car and I'm naked.'

The psychiatrist asks if I ever hear voices, if I have special powers, if I think about committing suicide. Eventually the interview ends. He confers with his colleagues. I am informed that I am to be discharged.

Very slowly, very carefully, I set off from the hospital on foot. Down the lane, around the corner, over the brow of a hill there are large meadows of common land, leading down to a golf course. I have never been to Wakefield before and I am lost. In the club shop I ask for directions and am sent back the way I have come, up over the hill, past the hospital and down into the town.

Weeks later, a ward manager will say, 'We knew you'd be back. The last thing we saw of you, you were stumbling around in the traffic.'

It is true I have problems with the traffic. For example, there is my system of identifying different cars. Steel-grey are special forces. White are government, blue are naval intelligence. Big black four-by-fours are military, and anything that catches my eye is covert surveillance. Then there is the problem of interacting with the drivers. I can't read their intentions. It's not clear to me if they will wait for me or whether I should give way to them. Sometimes I walk in front of them to prove they are watching me, and to make the point that I object to being watched and followed.

Scared and confused, I make my way into the town centre. First there is a large shopping precinct. I feel I should make contact with someone: in a vape shop a kind girl gives me a hit on one of her electronic cigarettes. Better. Now I am striding down into town, not quite lost as to what I should

do. I need to get back to Hebden. At the same time, I need
to be sure the security services have finished with me, that
my part is over. I want to know that my arrest and detention
worked like an airlock, a cleansing, that I am out. The interludes in the police station and the mental hospital seem
dreamlike and unbelievable, even now, the morning after, as
if they happened long ago. I decide to follow signs to the
Hepworth gallery. I have heard it is very good. I am longing
for something; I feel I will find it there.

'Horatio!'

I turn. It's one of my students from my time in Liverpool,
an excellent student, a good writer and a very kind person
who graduated the year I left. And here she is with her
parents.

'It's you!' she says. (Does she mean she knows something
about all this? The security services do recruit from universities . . .)

I shake hands with her mother and father. 'How are you
doing? Your work was so wonderful . . .'

'Good!'

'She's doing very well,' her father says, 'As long as she
gives up acting she'll be fine!' The family laugh. (By acting,
do they mean impersonation? Working for MI5?)

'What are you doing here?'

'I'm going to the Hepworth – do you know where it is?'

'Yes! You're on the right track,' she says.

'It's just down there, left, and right,' says her mother.
'You can't miss it.'

I thank them and we say goodbye and I hurry away,
convinced my student was expecting someone. She had obviously been told to look out for someone she recognised but
she did not know it was going to be me. The whole family
seemed to be waiting for something from me, and their directions were adamant . . . I am half reassured. That was a very
friendly contact. I am touched and more confused.

Abandoning plans for the Hepworth, I make for Wakefield Kirkgate station instead. There are signposts to a mosque. Should I follow them? Does my trail need to lead via a mosque? No. The station. Get home. Get to Hebden Bridge.

It is so very complicated at the station. There are lots of trains: I do not know if I should take a series of them and make a number of changes to throw off my pursuers or wait at the station for an indication of which I should take. I study the passengers. There is an anxious man with a rucksack, middle-aged and fit, who looks as concerned and confused as me. He is taking instructions from someone on his phone and looking at me, looking at the departure displays, hurrying from one platform to the other. There are discarded tickets on handrails and benches and around the ticket machine. Should I take them? What about DNA? Is this the crossing point, where my trail overlaps with the other man? I am exhausted by the anxiety of it all, by all the possibilities, by the plots and counter-plots. Eventually, beaten, I take a train to Leeds and another to Hebden. Home.

Rebecca takes one son to the station in the morning, does reading with the other, then takes him to school. She teaches online all day, picks up one from school, the other from the station, does the shopping, cooks the dinner, washes up, puts one to bed, attends to the other with whatever help he needs from school, hangs up the laundry, puts on the washing machine, finds time to feed and clothe herself, go running and exercise the dog – and then there is me.

'How did you do it?' I ask afterwards.

We stand in silence, the enormity of what she does and did between us, beyond words. She lets the silence answer, at first.

'You just . . . switch off,' she says.

And I know she has never switched off, not for a moment.

'All that and you were *teaching* too,' I protest. 'It's extraordinary.'

She laughs.

'The only reason I knew what had happened was because one of the policemen called me at five in the morning to tell me you had been taken to the hospital. He had stayed on over his shift and made them ask for another psychiatrist because you'd been saying you had taken drugs and the drug test had come back negative. But it takes longer to test for LSD and you seemed quite lucid. He said, "No, this isn't drugs, this is mental health," because he recognised you.'

But then of course Rebecca got a second call.

'I am very sorry,' the officer says, 'but they've let him go again.'

Not long after returning from Wakefield I make my way up the valley to the house. The boys are at school. Rebecca will not let me in. I was hoping to make up with her and have supper with them all: I post my shopping through the letter box.

It is icy cold. I go around to the back of the house where there is a spring and block the flow pipe. I want to make a sculptural waterfall of ice. I want to thank our neighbour, Lyndon, for being my overseer and trainer. I am sure he is ex-army and has taken on the job of bringing me on, of keeping an eye and an ear on us in our house. I want to watch the cars coming down our valley road. There are bases and safe houses in the wood; the great conference is over, all the VIPs are going back to their works and worlds. I stand at attention as they pass – let them see me, let them know how serious this all is, let them see someone who has been locked in cells and a mental hospital, has lost his family, son and house, all for the cause. Let them now do their part. It is time I got back to my other work.

I am supposed to be writing a children's book. I race through it, making wild changes. I need to make some money, rapidly. I send my agent and a friend in America, my former agent, a sheaf of documents, half-written books and fragments: how much will they give me for them? The box of books a publisher has sent me will be priceless, I know. I sign them, dedicating them to prime ministers, presidents and the finance minister of Nigeria. Worried questions and concerns are coming at me through the Internet from family, friends and contacts all over the world who have read my rantings on social media. Too much, too loud, too intrusive. I send vile messages to some of my friends – abusing Julien in Germany (I am sure he is a spy) and Evan in Canada (I am not even sure she is real). I know my laptop is stuffed with bugs, microphones, key-stroke loggers, viruses and hidden cameras. I throw it into the bath.

Along with everything else, Rebecca is dealing with the recovery of the car.

'The police couldn't tell me where the car was because you'd said you didn't want me to have any information. So then two weeks later the police get in touch and say, "The car's up at the reservoir, it's just off the road."

'So I went up to look for it and I couldn't find it so I rang the insurance company and went up there and met this lad with his little truck who was just there to pull a car off the side of the road. And we walked up and down and we couldn't find it. A police van happened to come the other way and the guy recognised me. He said, "Are you looking for your car, love? I'll show you." I said, "Is it just off the side of the road?" And he said, "Is it 'eck! I'll show you."

'I saw it and I said, "Are you fucking *kidding* me? After he did this, you let him go because he wasn't a danger to himself or others, after he did this?"

'He said, "I'm really sorry. We were all on your side, love, all of us."

'And the insurance company weren't going to cover it, they said they had to take it further, so the guy with the tow truck, who luckily really liked me, called his boss at the Star Garage and said, "This girl's in a real mess. If we don't get the car out she'll get done for polluting the stream." So he got it out – we had to get a tractor and tow it – and he brought it back here and let me get the stuff out of it.

'I got support from the police, but they were quite clear that the support they could give they gave on their own time.'

Ellie and Doug take my laptop to a shop – it is beyond repair. Ellie drives me to a rendezvous with Rebecca and our boy in a café. We both try not to cry as he climbs around on me and shows me toys. Rebecca is taking him to have a meal in the Tibetan restaurant. I could go with them. I think I am going to go, but instead I say I will get some tobacco and end up striding around the town, lost in the fantasy again.

Acting out a fantasy performs a therapeutic function, a kind of cracked and lived-out psychoanalysis. It might have taken months on the couch to establish what the delusions I have been playing out here made obvious. I long for significance, to play a role that matters in a life that has consequences. I want both to be an unseen mover behind the scenes – I was a very happy radio producer – and to be a star. I am an appalling egomaniac. I imagine that there are more things in earth and heaven than our familiar, consensual versions of reality allow. I long to touch the mysteries beyond the horizons, to commune with them, to be one with spirits and powers. Though I have built a life, some part of me wants to crash it into a reservoir, to swim free of it, to be renewed and reborn naked into the world. My frenetic need to be doing, to be acting, is easily explained. As Graham Greene comments in his essay 'The Revolver in the Corner Cupboard', about his games of Russian roulette, 'action has a moral simplicity that thought lacks'. The chaotic deeds of the insane are attempts to impose simplicity on the impossibly tangled consequences of our lives.

Everyone is trying, trying. I am trying too. I am trying to set in motion the creation of our great reward: a world school, based here in Hebden. Hebden Bridge is perfect for it, a kind, huge-hearted town. The place to begin is obviously right here, in my flat. We will need to knock through the east wall, where the shelves with the stereo stand. I move them and mark out the place. And we will need to make another door here, in the west wall of the pantry behind the kitchen, and one here, in the ceiling in the passage by the bathroom. I might as well set to it. I am about to when Philip and a doctor arrive.

'Come in! Come in! Do please sit down! Would you like some tea, some orange juice?'

I am elaborately courteous and deeply suspicious. What do they really want? To see inside my map room, the slit behind the bathroom? Let them.

They follow me on a tour of the small flat. They give little away; their actual role is to establish whether I have somewhere safe and suitable to live and to make a judgement about my fitness to remain in the community. My manner must be sufficiently plausible, because they leave.

Now my brother Alexander arrives. I am making a hole in the ceiling by the bathroom. It is harder than it looks.

'What are you doing?'

I take him outside and show him.

'You see? It all joins up. These flats are actually the basement of those houses, and if you link through there [a water tunnel, I think once a well, under the upper road], you can join them all up together.'

'Stop making holes in your ceiling!'

When he is not looking I push a five-pound note through the grating of a drain in the street outside. I try to reassure my brother. He buys lavatory paper for the flat and pizza for him. We go to see Zaff and have a relatively sane glass of wine.

Alexander is extremely gentle with me. He never confronts me with my madness; he seeks to make a calm place for both of us by trying to make sure I eat, by holding simple conversations with me, by making sure I take a sedative pill that evening, one of those prescribed by the doctor in Brecon over Christmas. He looks on as I show him the spaces between the bedroom floorboards and ceiling downstairs. This is the space I want to open in the ceiling outside the bathroom. He looks interested as I extract the magnet from the boiler system. I have thoroughly confused the electrics and the boiler by pulling switches and turning taps. Eventually I sleep well on the sofa bed in the flat's front room, insisting Alexander has the bedroom. He tells Rebecca and Doug that sleeping in the flat with me made for a terrifying night for him.

The next day, at last, they come.

CHAPTER 11

Sectioned

What a busy morning! Alexander goes out for coffee and supplies. I do some more banging and tearing at the ceiling; I am determined to break through today. Doug comes round and encourages me to discontinue the attack on the plasterboard. He makes no big thing of it. Rather, he looks at the damage, winces as you would at a child's mess and says, as if I am being unnecessarily silly, 'Stop now. You don't need to make a hole in the ceiling!'

'If you want a go, be careful, there's a razor,' I tell him. We are both staring up at the hole.

'Right. OK,' he says. 'Let's just leave it.'

Something about his manner, the good sense of it, the lack of alarm, disarms me. Fair enough. I will stop for the moment.

Now Rebecca comes round with her friend Jayn. Jayn is wearing suspiciously heavy, expensive glasses. It crosses my mind there may be cameras in them. I take them off her, look into her eyes and return them, still suspicious.

I am altogether fed up with the way people have been treating Rebecca, circling her, pursuing her. I am jealous. Her ex-husband paints pictures which look like her. They are very good and I have framed prints of them, but now I strip them from their frames, setting free Rebecca's spirit.

Now Vicky appears, another friend, and she and Rebecca are smoking cigarettes and laughing outside the front door,

which is open. People are coming and going downstairs.
Vicky has a lovely, funny and open manner, a Mancunian
directness and freshness. I decide I do trust Vicky.

I try to get on with the cleaning up.

'Here!' I say and drop a pole, a broken broom handle,
from the bedroom window on the first floor down to the
flower bed by the door. It lands next to Rebecca. She will
claim that I threw it at her, which is untrue, but the claim
helps, contributing to the decision which is coming.

What I want more than anything is to get my family back
together. To do this I begin to rearrange the bedroom: it
needs to be a pleasant space. Rebecca might want to work
here, or downstairs, so both areas need to be fit for her, with
books and desks.

I set it all up and light candles. It looks lovely. The day
is going quickly. Outside a police van has appeared, and an
ambulance. There are a lot of people downstairs now! Rebecca
and Vicky seem to be holding some sort of party. Tall men
in luminous jackets suggest I should go with them in the
ambulance. So does everybody. But I am the householder
here, I am appearing – certainly in my judgement – sane,
and so they cannot just manhandle me out of the door. I
could save everyone hours of bother and expense. I offer one
of the officers a copy of Bach. Laughingly, he refuses it. 'It's
going to be worth a lot of money!' I entreat him, but he is
firm. I scuttle back to my room. Let them mill around. They
all seem happy. Let them do their thing until they get bored
and go away.

Rebecca comes up and sits with me quietly on the bed.

'This is all for you,' I explain. She is unsettled, excited
somehow. I will calm her. I will calm everybody. I select
Andes by Michael Jacobs, a friend and hero of mine who
suddenly died a few years ago. He is one of my talisman
spirits; they form a small close family of the dearest dead
who I keep with me. I begin to read aloud. It is a fat book,

almost 600 pages. I will read it and read it until they all go away.

'Across unending grassland, towards evening. In a dented old taxi whose bonnet does not close properly. A tall man, squeezed next to the driver's seat, is being taken on an interminable straight road . . .'

It is the first peace we have had. Rebecca curls up on the bed for a little while.

I read on, but words can't keep it all back, cannot repel what is happening in the house or what is going to happen to me. I fall silent. Rebecca goes downstairs. She and Vicky appear and start to pack a bag for me. I cannot read now. Why are they doing that?

They go down again. I am not having anything to do with their plans. It is really time they went, along with their party.

My brother comes up. We sit for a while at the desk, a candle burning peacefully as we look out at the early dusk and the sky, the lights of windows and street lamps glowing on, the little town settling in for an early evening and a long quiet night.

'It's the perfect place for a study,' I say. 'It will be easy to work here, or for Rebecca to work here, if she wants to. It's just lovely with the view.'

If you look up, not down, you cannot see the police van and the ambulance, which seem to have been there for hours. Alexander sits so quietly with me. All the confusion downstairs seems held at bay, behind his back.

Many relatives must find themselves in my brother's position. Like my mother arguing both sides of my case – he is high but he is not dangerous, do not take him away – my brother wants me to be treated without being treated as a threat. A struggle has been going on out of my sight: Rebecca, Doug and Vicky have been telling him to call the police, to call the social worker, to demand, as a close relative, that I am assessed for sectioning. To make that case, he has to say

that I am a danger to myself or others. Alexander wants it
done gently: he calls the ambulance. Rebecca and Doug and
Vicky explain that the system does not work this way. The
ambulance crew cannot take me. The level of jeopardy has
to be higher. The nearest relative has to say more than they
want to say. There can be no mercy, no softening.

And now other people appear, besides the tall luminous
men in the living room. There are three: a lady, white, in
glasses. She might have stopped in on her way from the
shops; she carries no aura of power around her. A portly
Asian man wears a jacket and a professorial air. A very smart
young man, the same doctor who came the other day, carries
a laptop. They want to know if it is all right if they come
upstairs to talk with me. It is, of course. They are welcome.

Distressingly, I can only provide chairs for the lady and
the portly man, but the young man says he is fine standing
at the table. He is going to type a record of our conversation
on his laptop. I sit on the end of the bed. The lady leads.
She introduces herself and the men. She is a social worker,
the man beside her is a psychiatrist and the man standing is
a doctor.

Here we go again. I brace for battle. I know what to say
and how to say it – I mustn't talk fast; I mustn't become
agitated; no reference to any ideas or powers or projects;
nothing. Stick to the story. Listen politely. This is it: if I
can beat them I will be free, but if I make the tiniest slip
they will have me. Breathe.

'Can I offer you a cup of tea?'

The interview begins. It is just like all the others, only I
have a feeling of being extremely closely observed, and the
young doctor seems not to stop typing.

I give the same answers to the same questions. Eager to
mount the strongest defence possible, I say perhaps more
than I should. I do not come out with madness but rather
overdo the sane. The woman asks if I don't think it would

be best if I were to agree to go into hospital for a rest and treatment.

'I really don't need to. I can rest here.'

'Rebecca thinks you should. Your brother is worried about you. Your friends—'

'That really isn't my business. I am not responsible for their feelings. I am sorry they are worried or not happy or whatever, but this is a really important point that I've been working on with my therapist. She's very clear that it's important that I work on not taking responsibility for everyone else's feelings. I suffer from perfectionism, you see, I was told that in the Laura Mitchell centre in Halifax back in March – this was when I got the guidance on seasonal affective disorder. I think the person there is called Naomi?'

They listen and watch. Howsoever little I try to say, they somehow manage to say less, which makes me feel I am saying too much. Only the psychiatrist and the social worker ask questions. The young doctor looks at me and types and types.

'Can you tell us why you have been making holes in your ceiling?'

'Oh! Well. It's the roof space, right? It belongs to me. The flat has a problem with damp: by putting a ventilation hole there it helps the airflow, which really makes a huge differ- ence. It's just DIY. I don't think it's a crime . . .'

There are questions about the car crash, about being naked on the moors in the night; I give the answers which worked for the police and worked in the discharge interview. I must, surely, have done more than enough to satisfy them by now. I must have done enough to be free.

'I'm not sure what you want with me, to be honest. Do I seem mad to you?'

'Well,' says the psychiatrist, at last, 'you don't seem mad to me, no.'

'We will go downstairs and consult,' says the woman. 'And then one of us will come back up.'

After a while I go downstairs. The atmosphere has changed. There is an excitement among the press of tall, fluorescent men. I can feel them almost laying hands on me. The social worker approaches. Rebecca is with her.

'We have discussed the situation and we feel—'

'But you said someone was going to come upstairs.'

'But you came down! For your own safety, you are going to be taken to hospital, where you can be properly assessed and looked after. I have made an order to detain you under Section 2 of the Mental Health Act.'

'Who are you?'

'I am a social worker.'

'Can I see your ID?'

She shows me.

'This picture isn't even you. It doesn't look anything like you!'

'I had a different haircut.'

Two large men approach.

'I'll come with you,' my brother says. Doug has already volunteered to come with me. Everyone seems to want to come with me in the ambulance.

'Let me see your identity cards, please.'

The two large men hand them over.

'These are fake,' I declare and toss them up onto a high shelf. 'I'm going upstairs to get my bag,' I say. The game is up, palpably. Any second now they are going to grab me and cuff me.

I make it upstairs. Men in bulky jackets follow me. I drop my trousers and squat on the lavatory.

'What's he doing?'

'He's going to the loo.'

There is no lock on the bathroom door. One of them stands, looking in. No putting it off and nowhere to run. I wish I had finished the hole in the ceiling – I'd be through there and out of the house upstairs and into the woods, and they would never catch me.

'OK, that's it, time to go. Right now, please.'

I am wearing a pair of Doug's Crocs, corduroy trousers which are too small for me, an old shirt, a shabby jumper and an old coat. I have cut my own hair into a rough bob with bits sticking out. My bag has a random assortment of old clothes. So equipped, I climb into the ambulance. My brother gets in by the driver.

'I went before you left,' Doug says months later. 'When it was finally going to happen I didn't want to watch it really. I didn't see you being put in the ambulance. When we knew it was going to happen I left. I didn't want to see it.'

Doug is the most witty, giving man. Laughter follows him. He maintains an approach of enthusiastic apprenticeship to the world, meeting it with assurance and endless curiosity, eager always for its next folly, its next question or idea. He likes people inordinately and cannot help but let them know. Over the weeks of the crisis and the months that followed he and Ellie were inexpressibly kind to me and Rebecca. They made the difference throughout this story, supporting Rebecca, babysitting our boy, softly and carefully mediating between us, doing for us both whatever they could. Their house is a second home to dozens of us, their fortunate friends. Their wedding dissolved into riotous laughter whenever anyone tried to sum up Ellie. 'ALL RIGHT!' she cries when she sees you, whether she has stepped off a plane from China – where she was responsible for producing a TV history series in Mandarin, not one word of which she speaks – or just returned a gaggle of boys from Playtopia in Todmorden. She calls Doug Dougalicious.

Dougalicious has settled us at his kitchen table. We have small glasses of white wine. Typically, because he is a wonderful writer and an ever-thoughtful friend, he took notes at the time.

'I thought it might be helpful for you,' he says with a grin.

His house is close to the flat. The day I was sectioned he had been up and down, in and out all day.

'There were ambulance, police, a lot of people. They were there for ages – most of the day.'

'It seemed like a real party down there,' I say. 'The flat was full.'

'It was!'

'So . . . can I ask you what it was like? What I was like?'

'Yep. I've got my notes . . .'

He has his laptop out. He scrolls through screens.

'The thing that struck me – you were so in the moment. You were so *happy*. Whether you were cutting holes in your ceiling . . . I almost didn't want to stop you, though there was some talk of there being razor blades up there . . .'

'I was using a razor to pull the plasterboard down from the inside, the T-shape . . .'

'Ah right. You were so content! Like a young boy having a really good time. I almost felt at times I didn't want to jolt you out of that – in the short term – because you were so utterly content in the moment. But you were untethered and unmoored. Then you had that great craze of hiding five-pound notes in the drain – you told Ellie you could put chewing gum on sticks and fish them out – get rid of banks, you said!'

We laugh.

'Then there was setting up a book store on the street . . . I thought at the time it was like a shedding and a getting rid – an unburdening.'

That was the box of copies of the Bach book I left by the bus stop the schoolchildren use, with a note saying help yourself.

'At Christmas you went out and bought ludicrous things and gave them away – you were giving stuff to Zaff – you kept giving Zaff presents – you came over to us and gave us presents – a little picture frame, a Land Rover badge which I've got somewhere . . . But at certain moments it was like a religious experience; you were just getting rid of things, you were like the holy fool, the holy madman that you get in Tibetan Buddhism. You'd make very perceptive comments and you'd think he's *got through*, he's got through to another area, and there were really quite dark moments. Like when you were sitting by the fire and getting hot and you were talking about your sister and you said, "Say goodbye to my son," and we thought . . .

'At times you were so in that moment, and had this quiet restlessness, and kindness, I didn't see any nastiness, but then you'd flip from one idea to another. On Christmas Eve you were listening to yourself on the radio – at some level I could see that was slightly confusing – listening to this very rational version of you . . . Then there was – "Sugar cubes and Shakespeare," I've written here. Not sure what that means. And I've written things from Rebecca. She said you were pushing fish and condoms through the letter box.' He laughs awkwardly.

I say, 'I did do that. I'd been shopping and she wouldn't let me in. I mean, the fish was in a packet . . .'

'Oh right. You definitely needed booze – you took me to that hidden spot on the lane overlooking the town, then you pulled out brandy, whisky. We went to Nightjar and there was that nice Welsh barman and you got locked into conversation with him . . . Then you were wandering – sometimes I'd see you, or I'd hear afterwards you were wandering around Hebden. You told me later you'd seen Ben Myers and he'd given you money around that time.'

I exclaim, 'Oh God, yes, he did. I'd forgotten that. That was when I thought I was on E, when I thought I was testing out drugs to be legalised – it was herpes medication I found on the street near your house.'

'Yeah. So you were very much in the moment until you got restless or locked into very intricate stories. It was so lucid and so detailed. You always had an explanation – you said you were on acid, with the car, several times, though it wasn't clear where you got it from, but I knew you'd had some kind of psychotic episode . . . The way you behaved was an amplified version of some of the things you do or want to be – you did lose the sense of people around you. Normally you're good at gauging people around you, but you'd meet someone and go into hyperdrive.

'It was so hard to get you sectioned. It was really awful for Rebecca. You were clearly accelerating towards some kind of abyss or oblivion. I could see that if you carried on something was going to happen. But what you would do, very skilfully – I saw it on the day you were sectioned – was talk very rationally. You knew what to say. You'd slip into this mode, it was very manipulative. Alexander was very stressed by it.

'The person who was most useful in practical terms was Vicky – she was talking to the ambulance people and she knew what to say to them. They couldn't drag you down – until you acquiesced there was nothing they could do. Alexander and were I trying to coax you down. We started thinking, *Fuck, what does he have to do?* He's crashed his car, he's been taken into hospital and he's got out again; he's clearly going to have to do something really bad to himself. Your toe was going septic, you'd dropped your laptop in the bath. It's really hard to get socks in Hebden, it turns out but, I got you some socks – you weren't bothered about that or your toe. In some ways it was quite illuminating. These things don't matter. I don't want any socks! I don't care about my toe! That was the main worry: at what point would it go too far? What did you have to do? What became clear was that our perception of self-damaging and damaging to others was not the same as the ambulance people's. It's really tick-box.

The people were wonderful but the system is insane. I said to them, "You're saying people have to cause damage to themselves or use certain trigger words?" I remember Vicky and me saying, "He knows! He knows what not to say . . ."'

In the back of the ambulance with me is a tall, tired paramedic who is in fact the actor Tom Wilkinson, and a small policeman, a young man in his twenties. A lot of the policemen I meet during these weeks look like small actors in over-large luminous costumes. I guess we are going to do a programme, a BBC radio show recorded in front of a live audience. The policeman has a gently humorous air.

'How long have you been a stand-up comedian?' I ask.

'I'm not a stand-up comedian.'

'You can play with these buttons,' says Tom Wilkinson, impersonating the paramedic. There is a panel of switches to my left. Because he has invited me to, I do. Sometimes I sleep, though not for long. I pick up a cone of cup-like cardboard objects, like tiny bowler hats.

'Anybody want a hat?'

We might as well get into the comic spirit. I pass two through to the front for Alexander and the driver.

I wonder if we are in fact going to an airfield, in order to fly to London. I have the impression that my father is going to be at the National Theatre and I think we might be on our way to him.

CHAPTER 12

First night

'Here we are,' says the paramedic. Wet tarmac, dirty street lighting, glass doors. I know this place; this is the hospital in Wakefield again.

'I'm going to hold your arm now,' says the comedian-policeman, and he does, taking a very firm grip of my right bicep. Is he expecting me to act up? Very well, I will act up. I loll and reel, pretending to be drunk, singing, 'What shall we do with the drunken sailor / What shall we do with the drunken sailor / What shall we do with the drunken sailor early in the morning?'

As we enter the reception area we pass two men sitting slouched in chairs in front of a coffee machine. One is young, in his early twenties. Shaven-headed, he wears a grey track-suit. His face is heavy-featured and his expression thick with a kind of slow contempt. He looks at the policeman escorting me with a truculent hatred. The other is much older, a big man wearing dark clothing and a woollen hat pulled down low over eyes that are hard and still. He scares me.

'You will need codes to get out of the car park,' I tell my escorts, picking printed strips out of the box at reception and handing them over.

'It's fine, H,' my brother says, as we pass through a second door which locks behind us. 'It's just like the Metal Festival, remember?'

I did a turn at a festival by the Thames and invited him there.

'What do you mean?'

'Well . . . you remember. We stayed in that Premier Inn together. It's just like that.'

That helps. I've been here before and talked my way out of here before. Perhaps Alexander is right: perhaps it is just another stage in the festival game. There does not seem to be anyone around. There is an empty games room. I get out a table tennis net, stretch it half-heartedly across the corridor, think about coming up with some sort of game, abandon the idea and put it all back. My brother watches. There are biscuit wrappers and crumbs all over the canteen tables. I start clearing them up. Now I am in a storeroom signing a paper. My tobacco, money, lighter and belt are locked away. Now a nurse appears. Alexander speaks with him, says goodbye to me and goes. The paramedic and the policeman have gone too. Here is the family visiting room where I had my discharge interview, a miserable place. I hide a copy of my Bach book under one of the stools. Perhaps it will cheer someone up.

The nurse says his name is Ben. He is tall, young, deeply gentle and sympathetic.

'I would like a discharge interview, please.'

'Well the thing is, you are here under Section 2 of the Mental Health Act. I can't give you a discharge interview. You have to be seen by the senior clinician, who is a psychiatrist.'

'Can I see him now, please?'

'I'm afraid not. It's Saturday night. He won't be in until Monday.'

'Well can you call him?'

'I'm afraid I can't.'

'Why not?'

'I don't have his number. We don't call him out of hours.'

'But I shouldn't be here. I don't want to be detained.'

'I'm really sorry, Horatio. But you're here under Section 2, so you have to see the doctor.'

'Can't I appeal?'

'You can, yes.'

'I'd like to appeal now, please.'

'That's fine; I can do that for you.'

'When will we hear back?'

'It won't be till Monday that they get the paperwork.'

'I've got a lot of friends on newspapers. If I am going to be held here against my will I'm going to call all of them.'

'You are welcome to call anyone you like,' Ben says.

I think about it. 'But you'll put the appeal in now?'

'I will, yes. I'll put the appeal in for you.'

It seems unlikely that the nurse is going to do a sheaf of paperwork in the middle of the night. I have no idea what time it is; it feels like after midnight, but given I was taken into the ambulance just after dusk it must be around seven o'clock now. But I do trust him. He has a soft Liverpudlian accent and the most calm and gentle manner. He looks at you as though he hopes to understand you and believes that he does, or will.

'Thank you.'

'So what happens now is I'll show you to your room and we'll give you a check-up. Do you have any injuries or conditions we should be aware of?' he asks.

'I hurt my toe, it's swollen up. Otherwise I'm fine.'

'We'll have a look at that for you.'

In my room the door to the shower has sloped corners, so that you cannot get a ligature over it. There is plastic coating on the window, with a blowing-dandelion design. There is an overhead light which casts a stark yellow pallor. There is a plasticky under-sheet and duvet cover, a desk, a chair and warped plastic mirrors, guaranteed to make anyone look mad.

Imagine it's a hotel, I think. I've definitely stayed in worse. Whatever you do, don't ally yourself with the others. You are not a patient. You are a writer. You are not meant to be here. As soon as your appeal goes through you will be gone. You could be let out any minute. Act as though you belong to the world and you will soon be back in it.

'Do you have any laundry that needs doing?' asks a gentle man. He has steady eyes. His name is David. How calm he is! It puts me off my stride. He does not seem to want anything of me.

I might as well do a wash. Travel writing teaches you to do your laundry whenever you can. Travel writing. Right. That's what this is.

The laundry reminds me of the washrooms on ships I have sailed on, though the equipment is better. I put in a shirt, socks, a coat. Damn, though, was that a mistake? I can't go until they're dry. Never mind, the drier looks very good. I'll hit it up to the max and I'll be out of here in no time. The instructions seem simple but there is too much information and David is watching.

'Here,' he says mildly. 'See? It works like that.'

It's a ship-hotel and I am just passing through. That's good. I yaw about, waiting. People around the pool table ask who I am. One has long white hair and a Druidic air.

'I'm Stephen,' he says. 'Are you all right, mate?'

'I'm Horatio.'

'Horatio! What a name! That's a real name, isn't it?'

'Well it's a good name for a writer. I'm a writer.'

'Are you? Ah! We're both artists, you and me. I'm a musician!'

'Are you? What sort of stuff?'

'Dub-reggae. My band, we've toured everywhere – we're on the festival circuit . . . What do you write?'

How intensely he looks at me. What love he has.

'I can show you . . .'

I go back to the family visiting room, retrieve the book from under the stool where I hid it and show it to him.

Stephen is delighted. He shows the book to the men around the pool table.

'This is a really beautiful book,' Stephen says. 'We're real artists! You are. I am. I shouldn't be here, Horatio,' he says suddenly. 'I shouldn't *be* here!' His eyes fill with tears. Then he changes. 'You definitely shouldn't be here. You don't belong here, Horatio.'

For flashing seconds I know with certainty that he does belong here, and if he belongs here, then . . . I back away. My laundry is done. I shift it to the drier.

Ben the nurse calls me to the surgery. I apologise for the spectacle of my toe, which is disgusting. He takes a careful look and says that it is healing – worth monitoring but no immediate action required.

'So you're down to have two meds,' he says. 'A sleeping pill and quetiapine.'

'I don't take sleeping pills.'

'That's fine. You can choose not to take it. But you have to take the other, I'm afraid. I have to see you take it.'

'What if I refuse?'

'We really don't want to go down that route. It can be given intravenously . . .'

'What is it?'

'It's an antipsychotic.'

He lets me see a leaflet, densely written in small type, listing dozens of side effects. I don't want to be held down and injected. I take it. I retrieve my laundry and yaw about again.

I am in the day room, looking at the bookshelf by the pool table, when suddenly my legs are groggy and my vision spirals. I feel sick. The floor seems to undulate and tilt. Dizziness hits me like a wave. My hearing goes funny.

'Look at him, the poor bastard,' says an athletic young man in shorts by the pool table. 'That's the serotonin, draining out of him . . .'

Quetiapine has thrown a blanket over the D2 receptors in my brain. The synaptic receptors, accustomed to a manic tide of serotonin and dopamine, are suddenly denied. Now they scream for their fix. It feels as though I am hurtling towards semi-consciousness. I weave to my room and crawl into bed. I half-sleep as if in a storm, drenched and plunging through sweat and rushing, falling sensations, awaking feverish, going under again. I do not know what time it is when I make it back to the nurses' station, the corridor undulating.

'I want to report a bad reaction,' I say. I am very upset.

This is a terrible place. Thank God I will be leaving tomorrow. Later again I get up and take my bag to the office. I have woken with the absolute conviction that this is a ship-hotel. And there's David by the office.

'I'm going to leave my bag here,' I tell him. 'I'll collect it from reception before I go.'

'You can leave that, sure,' he says easily.

CHAPTER 13

First day

There are iron shutters on the windows with small holes in them, so that if you unfocus your eyes you can see through them quite clearly. There is a small car park out there, and a stack of Portakabins. A tired thought suggests that the cabins are where they are operating now, my watchers. There are men coming and going, eating bacon sandwiches in a van. They look like builders.

'Breakfast!'

Out of our rooms we come. There is a man who looks as though he has escaped from a film, his hair cut wildly and standing on end, his eyes staring with unregistering frankness, skin sheened with chemical side effects; he wears a shambling tracksuit. There is Stephen, beautifully apparelled in a bright smock, many-coloured, perhaps South American, and smart clean jeans. He smells of the shower and soaps; he is businesslike and hearty, as though we are all on a residential art course and he is a tutor.

There is the athletic boy, James, in shorts and some sort of football shirt, who looks more normal than any of us – entirely normal, in fact, alert and sunny. One of the loudest of us is a man in black. Yorkshire-accented, he wears a wool beanie, bounces with energy, stands very close to you, studies you with quick eyes, shakes hands. 'Jason,' he says.

There is a silent man whose gaze is turned entirely inward, as though he does not see you in order that you might not see him. He sits alone, looks uneasy if you catch his eye. He turns his gaze to the tabletop as if reading it.

Joshua comes in, swaying slightly, walking very slowly. He seems lost in a different dimension. He looks out with a gaze which seems somehow torn, as if he has become confused somewhere off to the side of reality, as if he can see it but cannot quite return to it. It is as if he is almost able to hear, and only just unable to speak. He seems mystified and oppressed by whatever his senses are telling him. When the staff talk to him they do it loudly. Much of his life is spent walking the corridor very slowly, talking to himself, his lips moving, eyes distracted.

Breakfast is served through a hatch. Toast is made for us by Yorkshire ladies with matter-of-fact expressions. They treat us as though we are sane. I try to show sanity. Show sanity. Make the instant coffee without spilling any of the powder. Get the cereal out of the boxes without making a mess. Pour the milk without splashing. Get it back to the table, with the wrapped butter pat and the capsule of jam, without a hesitation or an error. They are watching.

There are four this morning, two men and two women, sitting along the window, about a yard from the nearest tables. They say good morning to us and we to them. They are staff – nurses, support workers; I do not know what everyone does, except that they watch us.

I have never eaten under formal observation before. It feels a strange and quixotic task. Can you spread butter on cool toast sanely? Stephen and James the sportsman talk cheerfully. I am slow, my thoughts syrupy. I want to go back to bed. You can finish breakfast as soon as you like but I figure you want to demonstrate a healthy appetite.

The staff talk in a desultory way. Behind them the light brightens in a yard. It is going to be a sharp clear day. I want to ask about my appeal. I want to do something that contributes to progress, to getting out of here, but the ward is sluggish this Sunday morning. Patients wait around outside the glassed-in office. Staff type and exchange comments inside. There is something inevitably reminiscent of zombie films in the way we hang around, watching them, waiting.

On the wall is a chart of all the staff, faces, names, a line or two about each of them: 'My name is Jade and I like baking cupcakes!'

I study the faces and the names, trying to memorise them. It feels like the first test of the mad – can you distinguish sane people who work here from mad people who do not? It is harder than it looks. Is it really a test? I do not know anything. Further down the corridor are large printed sheets about our rights as sectioned patients. I read them and read them but it is hard to make them stick. People who can release me include my 'responsible clinician' and my 'nearest living relative', who may not be a relative.

I have the right to appeal and have my case heard by a tribunal. I have the right to a legal advocate. A list of qualified local lawyers specialising in these cases is available.

The power seems to reside with the deputy ward manager, Nigel, a man with white hair and glasses, a large rangy frame and a restless manner, whose voice and accent are strong and certain and local. Nigel is preoccupied this morning and cross about something. I hear him shout at one of the staff. I want to know when I can meet my responsible clinician, I want to know when I can get out of here. Get out of here. Get out of here. Don't say it. Don't think it. Even through the wooze it is clear I would be crazy to claim I am sane.

'You're on the list to see the doctor,' Nigel says.

I drift around the ward. We are in a low, white building, new-looking. It has twenty-two rooms arranged in an angular figure of eight around two inner yards. The yards have AstroTurf in the middle. Around the edges are flower beds strewn with woodchip and haggard clumps of lavender. There are tables and chairs in the bigger yard and a view of the sky. If you stand in one corner of it you can see part of a treetop.

As well as the bedrooms, there is the dining room with its serving hatch to a food prep area and internal windows giving on to the smaller of the yards. There is an art room, which is not large but richly equipped with different kinds of card and paper, pens and paints. There are two small games rooms, one of which has a PlayStation, the other a large TV.

We share the dining room with patients from the women's ward. They eat before us, the door on our side of the dining room locked, so that we never overlap.

The main room we frequent is a large day room with a huge high-definition TV at the far end and a pool table near the door. Between them are large sofa-chairs in rows facing each other. There is a very small bookshelf – I can see one Philip Pullman, a Lee Child, two Rosamund Pilchers and a single Flashman.

A single window in the corridor overlooks a car park, a hedge and a low roof, and beyond, the spire of Wakefield cathedral and a wooded ridge in the distance. The window has a deep ledge you can sit on.

Now it is time for meds. The men line up or come and go from a ragged line outside the surgery.

Stephen is in there a long time. He bursts out now, terribly distressed, and strides away to his room, crying and ranting. They are out to get him. They are not listening to him. They are trying to mess him up, to force him, to poison him. They are not listening.

I am not down for meds. I circle the bookshelf, pick out the Flashman, the Reacher and Philip Pullman's *The Ruby in the Smoke*. I hoard them in my room. In the art room I pick out paper, too thick and expensive for writing paper really, but it will have to do. On my bed I open the Flashman and try to concentrate. Abyssinian history. I cannot tell if it all has significance or if it is all meaningless. I should be working. If am reading then I am working. If I am working then this book has meaning for me, only I cannot follow it.

I retrieve my bag from the office but do not unpack it, determined not to be here long, determined not to settle in. The bag will live on the lower shelf nearest the door. The clothes I have with me are shabby and awkward: trousers that are too small, old checked shirts, an odd top. The Crocs are ridiculous, though perfectly practical for the ward. I am unshaven and dishevelled. For some reason I have very smart new socks . . . Doug! Doug got me new socks. My eyes water. God bless him.

But what now? Friends, contacts, moves, plans . . . *Come on!* You used to be a BBC producer. You have been trained to handle more or less anything, organise anything, get results. But you have no computer, no phone; your money was taken and they are very careful with the locked doors, two of which separate you from the car park. Looking at the larger courtyard, you can see how the drainpipes could be used to reach the roof. Climb one and you would quickly be one storey up, escape certainly feasible. But they would be on you in minutes – you'd be lucky to make it to the golf course . . .

By 10 a.m I am back in bed.

I sleep fitfully for an hour and get up, full of plans formed in thin dreams. Paper, pen. You are a writer; what else do you need? I start drafting an article I was supposed to be working on. See? I don't have to be a lunatic in an asylum. I can be a journalist. I was in Italy in the autumn, staying in Francis Ford Coppola's villa, and I haven't written it up. I write a first paragraph. It's too lurid, too opaque somehow. 'An aeroplane on approach to Bari, the Sirocco blowing out of an orange sunset, warm mist swirling over the coast . . .' It's wrong. It's clichéd. I cross it out and try again. Better.

But my thoughts are muddled, there are too many of them and they won't stick to the paper in order. More crossing out. Back to bed. Read Lee Child. I love Jack Reacher normally, but this one feels exhausting, full of troubling references. I cast it aside. I sleep again, for fifteen minutes. I wake and nothing has changed, except that the first five minutes of waking seem to brim with optimism and plans. What to do? Get up and out and circle the ward.

The same figures are hanging around the staff office, attracting the same glances from the staff inside. There is an air of vague wanting and indeterminate waiting. Constant daytime junk splays across the huge TV on in the day room. High definition makes it look too real, not like TV at all, as though it is a window on to a collection of actors in slapped-on make-up performing awkwardly in a room next door. I drift into the art room. There are red and blue painted signs in here, recently completed, messages of hope and encourage-ment in the same kind of tone I remember from working in prisons. WE ARE STRONG [honestly, we are], WE ARE HERE, WE WANT TO BE BETTER, WE WILL BE BETTER . . . I turn away, feeling sick. They won't catch me in here, painting away the days of my life in sunny slogans. I go out to the larger exercise area. It is cold under a raw sky. I circle it, pacing. Exercise, that's right: get fit, stay strong, walk.

You cannot walk for long in circles, it turns out. It feels too desperate and it must look mad from the office. Back inside, back to the room, back to the draft I go. It's all crossings-out. Hopeless.

As the confines of this ward release me from booze, drugs, lack of food and sleep, my first day (and many to come) is shot through with flashes of agonised uncertainty. How can I explain that first contact thing on the Internet? What about the conversation with Natasha and Chris? What about the Dolomites? I flinch and cringe internally at every recalled moment. The past and the outside world conflate into a whirl of confusion and shame. Without the delusions, the unbearable enormity of what I have done is a giant hammer hovering over me and everyone I love. The madness offers to hold it off, to dissolve it, but every time I think of something I did I feel revolted and exhausted.

I sense but do not yet know how fortunate I am. This ward is calm, clean and well run. I do not know that some of the key nursing staff are cracking under the strain of the administration they must do, the lack of backup available to them and the frustration they feel, daily, at not being able to spend time with patients, to try to understand and help us.

The worst room on the ward is brightly lit and bare but for a single chair and a payphone which works sometimes. It reminds me of boarding school, of being far away from home and not in control. I call my mother and beg her to help me get out. She refuses. 'You need help,' she says. My father says the same thing. 'They know what they are doing.' Rebecca is unshakeable. 'You need to get a proper assessment,' she says. I talk to my son. I tell him I am fine. I tell him I love him. I will see him soon. He tells me he is fine. He tells me he loves me. I hope he thinks I am away on a travel writing job. Rebecca gives that impression but I am not sure. He will be six on Wednesday. It is now Sunday night.

Because Sunday lunch is substantial, Sunday supper is junk. Dismal sandwiches, crisps, bits of pizza and sweet things. I found it hard to characterise the atmosphere of those evening meals at the time, something odd about it, something amiss – but I think now I know what it was. Emptiness. Sunday night all over the Western world is slightly nostalgic for the weekend gone and somewhat braced for Monday. But not here, not in the mental hospital. We have meetings, hopefully, scheduled with the psychiatrist. We may have visits to look forward to, if that is the phrase; some of us may have release hours or days coming up. We all have our regular schedule of medication to face, tomorrow morning and evening, and every morning and evening, and in that we are no different from any patients in any hospital anywhere. We can now tick off another day lived and behind us, another step, another number on our charts.

For some of us the magic number is twenty-eight: for those on Section 2, twenty-eight days means release or re-admission – either way, it is a significant moment. Why, then, the emptiness, the feeling of stasis? Because, I think, in the rock bottom of most of us there is a feeling that even if the surface conditions are improving, in that the days and hours of our detention are passing, in our hearts we know, or have been led to believe, that nothing fundamental is going to change. Our brains are ill. Nothing is going to alter that. The fact that we are here is proof that we are almost as ill as it gets. (There is an intensive-care ward, for the worst afflicted, where some of us have been.) One or two of us, heads bent under the yellow light, will be here, doing this, feeling this way, a year from now or more. Much, or something, anyway, may happen in the coming week, but in the end, this is us – dishevelled men eating crap sandwiches under yellow light, watched by tired staff, in a mental hospital.

We chew our food and stare into space, mostly lost in our own thoughts. Later there is the meds queue. There is some pool-playing and some television-watching, until one by one we head for our rooms, our beds and whatever sleep our conditions and medications allow. It is a broken sleep because we are checked every hour. Our guardians need to see move-ment from us. Through the glass panels in our doors they shine a torch at our eyes until we react.

CHAPTER 14

Day 2

Sunrise is cold and lancing, the car park beyond the window steaming with frost-mist and the sky freezing, raked with the first jet trails. At breakfast I sit with Stephen and James, the young athlete. Stephen is often ebullient, talking and talking, incredibly generous in his assessments of you and anything you say to him. Everything you come up with is true, everything you suggest or conclude is brilliant. He is a musician, well read and much travelled, having toured with his band. He is very proud of Wakefield – 'Wakey'. He struggles with emotion. He feels things keenly and gets worked up very quickly.

'We're all geniuses here!' he cries. Indignation at our treatment, assertion of our worth and hopelessness at our prospects are a turmoil within him. His pale blue eyes fix yours and he talks passionately, pleading to the world through you.

'They won't listen to me, Horatio, they just won't listen to me. I shouldn't be here! You shouldn't be here! Anyone can tell, we shouldn't be here, and they won't fucking listen to me, and they keep giving me these pills that fuck me up . . .'

If you have a streak of conservatism in you, Stephen will bring it out. I feel that I should be here, and Stephen should be here, whether or not they are listening to him, which of course they should be.

Delighted laughter and furious tears take turns to possess him. When he clashes with the nurses over his medication his distress is awful to witness. He sobs and curses furiously, he storms away along the corridors to his room.

But when Jason takes a bad phone call Stephen is with him instantly, his arm around Jason's shoulders.

'You're all right, mate, you're all right, mate,' he says, hugging swarthy Jason tightly. 'It won't be like this for ever, it won't, it won't.'

When one of us is upset Stephen and James are often the first to react. They offer pats, hugs, reassurance, solidarity. They are the first among us, somehow, the McMurphys of this Cuckoo's Nest.

James might have escaped from a boys' comic from the last century. He is all ripples and triangles, toned muscle. His hair stands up in a kind of quiff and his face would fit in a strip-cartoon about Spitfires, bright with the openness and innocence of the football hero, honest and ready to smile. It turns out his game is rugby. He plays to a professional standard. We begin to get to know each other around the pool table, which is the heart of the ward.

'Because of the way my system's imbalanced I actually need amphetamines – you know, speed! – to slow me down, to balance me out. You can tell by how fast I talk, can't you, that's the problem, so they're trying to sort it out, because otherwise I get really bad anxiety, like *really bad* like I can't do anything, but that being quick is who I *am* too, if you get what I mean? Like fast in life, fast in speech and thought!'

We start to talk about rugby – he often carries a ball around, tossing it from hand to hand – and then we end up outside, passing it, while James demonstrates feints, dummies and sidesteps, talking at top speed, if not perhaps top speed for him, about his playing career and his hopes and his parents and his troubles: 'I were smoking a lot of weed, skunk, like,

a lot of weed, because it brings me down, but it's no good
for you, is it? Fucks you up and makes you paranoid, so what
I've decided to do is just do the whole twenty-eight days
under Section 2, just do them, no appeals or anything like
that, so I can have a rest and they can get my medication
right and then hopefully I can go back to playing. I'll have
lost a lot of fitness but you have to try, don't you?'

It was James who made the comment about the dopamine
draining out of me when the quetiapine hit. He has studied
biology and physiology to undergraduate level as part of
sports science. He is fluent in receptors, synapses, transmitters. His sketches of how brain chemistry is affected by
cannabis, dopamine, serotonin, amphetamine and antipsychotics are lucidly delivered at zipping speed, his hopeful
and searching gaze on you as he talks. James' intensity
reminds me uncomfortably of me in my mania. Listening to
him, I experience something of the unease that those around
me must have felt, dealing with me. I find myself talking
slowly in reply, trying to slow him down.

'You can tell – I can see it in you, mate! I can see it by
the way you're reacting that I'm too fast, aren't I? A bit
manic like? That's because I haven't had my meds yet. I'll
get my meds and I'll be like – ahhh! They make me sleep
a lot though and the timing is really awkward because here
they do them twice a day, but if you look at the interval
and how long they last for and how long the effects take
to wear off I really need them in a different dose three
times . . .'

You could actually go mad, stuck here. I spend time on
the one windowsill in the corridor which has the view of
Wakefield cathedral spire and that wooded ridge, Woolley
Edge, beyond. I take short bursts of sleep. I pace the yards,
spotting birds and aeroplanes above them. God, I want *out*.
I beg and wheedle on the phone. No good.

'You need a proper assessment,' Rebecca repeats.

'You're being looked after there,' my mother says; you can hear her confirming it to herself, reassuring herself as she speaks.

'It will take time for them to find the right medicine for you,' she says.

I speak to my little boy and tell him I love him.

'Love you too, Dad,' he says, sounding dutiful and guarded.

I desperately want to be out in time for his birthday, the day after tomorrow. The paperwork on my appeal has gone through, say the nurses. I need to choose a mental health lawyer to make my case. Appeals have to be heard within fourteen days. I will have a meeting with my responsible clinician, they promise, though they cannot say when that will be.

Don't protest that you are sane, I think. *Be* sane. No sane person claims they are not mad. It feels like a sardonic and crushing catch-22. I'm going to have to be patient. I'm going to miss my boy's sixth birthday.

I reel from hope to grey despair. My fellow 'service users', as we are called, spend a lot of time going out for cigarettes. I am not smoking. I have fixed on this as something positive I can do, something I can take back to my boy in lieu of a missed birthday and no present. But it would be wonderful to stand at the door of the unit, in the car park, and feel normal for a moment.

And then suddenly – a visitor! Everything changes with the appearance of Chris, one of my oldest friends, who has come up from London. For a couple of hours we discuss a thousand things.

They let us roam about in the smaller of the two yards, which helps, as I hate the dining room. (We all hate the dining room with its yellow light and blank walls.) We talk about the time Chris spent in Rwanda, about his work and about Brexit: he is a passionate campaigner against it.

He seems thinner than the last time we met. He is wonderfully energised and invigorating company. We laugh and feel our way along webs of connection and history and friendship. He has a meeting, perhaps, with the shadow transport secretary tomorrow, he says. He is hugely involved in Active Transport, a movement to get people walking and cycling.

For all the quiet madness of our surroundings we are entirely at home in each other's company. 'Wakefield's probably a more interesting place to watch Brexit than Westminster,' he says when I say I wish I was on College Green. It seems so recently that Rebecca and I and our little boy were there, singing songs and waving flags with Extinction Rebellion.

Chris comes back after supper. On his iPad we watch May's attempt to pass a Brexit withdrawal bill defeated by an historic margin. While he is here it feels as though I am involved in the world again. He says many kind and sensible things. 'Get well, H. Take your time . . . There's no rush.'

He is right, of course. As he heads back to London I turn in, mulling. You could pretend you were here by choice, I think. You could try to accept it.

CHAPTER 15

Day 3

I wake happy. It feels as though I am sweating out the madness at night. Beyond my sliding window the sun is a fiery pearl. The observations last night, as every night, were hourly: each time they shine a torch in your eyes and watch you until you move. They seem to do this every fifteen minutes when they want you up in the morning, but that may be sleep-fuddled illusion. Before it got light, someone shone a torch in my eyes until I swore.

Shower. Teeth. Dress. I am less paranoid today that the various devices in the ceiling conceal cameras, though the wonky distorting mirrors are unhelpful. I say good morning to a patrolling member of staff. Her Wakefield accent is pleasing and funny.

It is the kind of breakfast I ate when I travelled with container ships – Weetabix, white toast, butter, jam. Not spilling anything and eating under the eyes of the staff is easier today. Not thinking about my family is harder. There are moments of terrible pain when I think of my little boy breakfasting, getting in the car, going to 'work', as we call his school run. I could hear him in the background of the phone call last night, talking to his brother, who was saying 'You can't watch that!' to him, gently.

Rebecca sounded calm. The dynamic between us is a turmoil of love, care, suspicion, hurt, fury, cooperation; how ten years of deep understanding can turn into a future of absolute unknowing. What will happen to *us*? We still love each other. Sometimes, these last months, I have felt we were so close that we thought as one. In dreams I seem to talk to her all the time.

I breakfast with my new friend Pete, who was a civil servant. He is a reader (the first, apart from Stephen, who has taken to the Bach book like a Bible) and he is into horses. Lester Piggot's autobiography, he says, is a good 'un. Three staff watch us eat. When they are aware they are being listened to they raise their voices self-consciously and talk about . . . steaks, this morning. One, an obese and friendly presence, claims that a king appreciated his steak so much he dubbed it 'Sir Loin'. Breakfast could not yield much better than this, I think.

'Your solicitor is here!'

The nurse doesn't quite exclaim it but you can hear the happiness in her voice. Bless them, they are all rooting for me. My solicitor is Sarah Cunnane LLB (Hons) of Switalski's Cheapside, Wakefield.

Talking to Chris last night was wonderfully reassuring, but with Sarah on my side I feel, for the first time, that I will leave here as soon as I rightfully should. She is an intense and hurried and focused woman who does a thorough interview with me at tremendous speed, writing everything down with fierce concentration. We will win the appeal, I am sure of it.

I feel terrible shame over the immense expenditure of time and effort I have cost the country, councils, the NHS and police. I keep saying sorry. But then, as everyone says when I apologise, 'It's what we're here for.'

Afterwards I go out and walk the decks, circling the yards in the cold air. I make to-do lists of the simplest things. I need my window opened, and to enquire about the possibility of swimming. I ask if I can have a haircut.

'In the next three weeks,' they say.

'I'll look like a hedge by then! Is it possible to go swimming?'

They look uneasy.

'There is hydro but you're not down for it. We'll see what we can do . . .'

I speak to Dad. He is worried, cold and angry. 'They've seen it a thousand times before,' he says. 'Do what they tell you.'

As yet they are not telling me to do anything. Everything depends on the responsible clinician, the psychiatrist Dr X. All of us are entirely in his hands. I should have had a meeting with him within seventy-two hours of arriving, yesterday, Monday. I will see him today, they say, later.

In the meantime I am making friends. James is adorable, so bright and sympathetic. Stephen and he are the only other Remainers I have met. Pete, with his straggly hair and sweet sad face, a long-term depressive, is an easy, natural friend, experiencing exactly the hell I remember in depression of wanting not to exist for his family's sake.

We talk about all sorts of things, including politics. Pete voted out of Europe. He says he would feel humiliated by another referendum and would relish an election: 'I'd feel respected,' he says. We are naturally tactile, touching each other's arms, hand-on-shoulder gestures, and easily amused. We discuss Thatcher. They hate her so much here that saying her name is like summoning Beelzebub. I do not fully understand the depth of their antipathy until I meet Arthur, a fellow patient. I think he is addicted to opioids. He has the most beautiful east Yorkshire accent. He calls me 'cock' or 'cocker', short for cockerel, I think.

He tells me his grandson has applied for twenty jobs. 'Not one interview. Wants to be a builder.'

Our conversation drifts until we hit on the miners' strike.

'Farmers ploughed fields for us so we could get tatties. Out picking, all of us, to feed family.'

'It must have been like a war,' I say, 'like refugees in a war?' He looks at me and nods.

We came in at the same time. 'Nothing wrong with being here,' he insists. 'Nothing wrong.' He came in on a stretcher – alcohol and morphine, I think. His family are visiting today. He talks about the fear and humiliation he feels at the prospect of them, and the delight at their appearance. Paranoia is our biggest foe, perhaps.

The locks and keys between us and the world seem to unleash terrifying visions. Last night, looking at my swollen ankles and thinking about my light head, I was halfway sure I had been on lithium since I arrived. (Only a tribunal will clear this up, I thought. Perhaps this has been the agenda all the while. For there are agendas, of course there must be – how does anything come into being without a process, a map, a flexible but firm and corporeal plan?)

I wait and wait to see Dr X, my responsible clinician. They keep telling me he is busy, will see me soon, that my name is on the list.

And then the afternoon wanes and they say no, he has gone. I am furious and stricken.

'But you promised! You promised all day. And I've been waiting and waiting.'

Ben, the nurse I like very much, can see how upset I am. And I can see that it is not his fault and that it would be wrong to take it out on him, and yet I feel betrayed, let down, played for a fool.

'So I can't see him? I can't call him? I can't do anything – you can't do anything?'

'I'm sorry, Horatio, I can't.'

'I am absolutely devastated. I was promised *all day*.'

'I really am very sorry,' Ben says, and I can see in his face that he is. And now I'm going to cry, for fuck's sake. I flee to my room.

Later I break. I ask for a nicotine substitute.

'Will this count against me?' I ask the nurse.

'Of course not!' she says. 'Have something, if it will make you feel better.'

CHAPTER 16

Day 4

'Is it possible I could have a shave?'
'Yes! We can do that. You need to be supervised, though. Can you give us about half an hour?'

The razor is a two-bladed Bic. I have rarely managed to use one without cutting myself but I am determined to pull it off today. Two of the support workers, both young women, are detailed to observe the operation.

Carefully, carefully I make a lather, mixing a squirt from the liquid soap sachet with a squirt from the shampoo sachet. There is a trick to everything. To prevent you drowning yourself or flooding the bathroom the tap over the basin is on a timer – it will run twice in succession for a few moments before it cuts out for ten minutes. The shower is on the same system, though it runs for longer.

The two women and I keep up an easy chatter as I shave, very carefully. Triumphantly uncut and smooth-jawed at the end of it, I return the razor to them and feel a surge of something like achievement. Survival in here is going to take routine. I think of my father, who was in an isolation ward for weeks this summer as he underwent chemotherapy for leukemia.

'They said I was the first patient they had ever had who got up every day and made the bed,' he told me. He devised a daily schedule of pacing his small room, listening to music, reading and correspondence. Now I make more to-do lists: shave, walk the yard, read, sleep, write, socialise. It would be a bad idea to withdraw entirely to your room even if you felt like it. You need to show you can interact normally with other people, however normal or otherwise they are.

Before lunch comes a phone call. It's Doug: 'We're four miles away!' Doug and Ellie. They have driven across Yorkshire to see me, bless them.

They arrive with the looks I have grown used to seeing on new faces in the ward: fear that it will be hellish, relief that it seems quiet, apprehension at how they will find you, comprehension when they find you apparently sane, caution when they place this in the context of what you have done and the fact you are here. We meet in the windowless family visiting room, under grim light. They are so quickly, wonderfully sunny, though we are confined to that awful room. They have brought my boots – the incredible pleasure of boots! And my terrible old coat, in which I danced in the New Year of 2005 in the Rif in Morocco. They say Rebecca is doing well and our boy is doing well and they are going to have pizza at his birthday party this evening. Doug offers to give him a present from me. I want to show them around but it is not permitted.

Later I speak with Dad again. He is hostile, suspicious, shaky. I read out a letter I wrote to him last night. It tries to explain that just as he has taken huge pride in my achievements he also takes my defeats and disasters personally, which cannot be good for either of us. He listens.

After lunch in the day room, Hector, the support worker who made the announcement at breakfast yesterday about the king knighting his steak, reveals himself to have been a tremendous pool hustler. For a while Hector and James and I knock balls around and talk. There is laughter and lightness: we might not be in a mental hospital at all. Then James offers me use of his laptop. I have to obtain permission to borrow it. Permission is granted. Joyful, I hustle to my corridor window. I have dozens of emails. There is time enough to deal with the top few. Then . . .

'Dr X wants to see you.'

And Jason wants to talk about writing, how you make a living. And the cleaners want to talk about a key. I return the laptop and enter the presence of Dr X, who is sitting in a room with a student, a quiet girl with a gentle air, which seems to leaven the atmosphere.

The famous Dr X seems calm and pleasant, as one would hope. He is very well dressed in herringbone tweed. He looks uneasy about something – perhaps his power, which throws the whole ward into a flurry of appeasement and speculation.

The matter of the interview is predictable. There is another rehashing of my decline and fall. But the manner is different again. In the corner Helen, fast Helen, a light-footed and quietly watchful manager – touch-types. I remember my mantra. I talk slowly. I try to think slowly. I tell the story I am asked for. I add only what they seem to want. I try to remember, above all things, that I am here to elicit information. (What is wrong with me? What do I need? How can you help? What do I need to do to get the help from you that I need?)

It is a delicate dance. If Dr X gets it wrong, I will pay. If he mis-prescribes, sending me down a chemical wormhole into a world of pills and side effects, requiring more pills and causing more side effects, that is tough luck on me. But if he gets it very wrong, he will answer to a coroner's court. For example, if taking the wrong pills drives me to kill myself, or he allows me to leave too soon or to take no pills, and I kill myself or someone else, it will surely come back at him.

I do not know what I was expecting: some kind of analysis, some kind of exploration, searching questions, perhaps. Instead, this crucial twenty minutes passes off as a piece of routine, with a non-conclusion.

Dr X seems to have everything he needs to know in front of him. It is as though he has summarised and concluded my case before meeting me. He asks how I am. He runs over my longitudinal history. He gives a lot of credence to Rebecca: I am not going to be released if she is not happy for me to come out, it seems. I talk about stress and cannabis and cyclothymia. Dr X is not interested. He instructs that I be given three sheets of paper on three possible pills: lithium, sodium valporate and aripiprazole.

The sheets are double-sided A4 produced by the NHS. They lay out what each drug does, some of their possible side effects, how long they need to take effect and what happens if you come off them.

Sodium valporate is used for epilepsy and bipolar disorder. You take it twice daily. Side effects include stomach aches, diarrhoea, weight gain, shakes, headaches, thinning hair, torpor, liver damage, suicidal thoughts and pancreatic damage. As to its efficacy, the NHS says, 'We don't fully understand how this medicine works for treating bipolar disorder. However, sodium valporate is thought to reduce or prevent manic episodes by increasing the amount of a chemical called gamma-aminobutyric acid (GABA) in the brain. GABA blocks transmission across nerves in the brain and has a calming effect.'

All well and good, I think, but I have never had a manic episode without adding cannabis to stress, so as long as I stay away from cannabis I am not worried about having one again, so I am not going to take this medicine.

Lithium I dismiss. There are too many reports of lithium placing a deadening screen between the user and the world. If I cannot write, I cannot live, and I am not sure I would want to live without writing. They can keep it.

This leaves aripiprazole. Again, how it works is unclear. Common side effects include difficulty with speaking, drooling, loss of balance control, muscle trembling, jerking or stiffness, restlessness, twisting movements of the body, uncontrolled movements (especially of the face, neck and back) constipation and disrupted sleep. Manic spending, sexual disinhibition and early death have also been ascribed to aripiprazole.

What do I do?

I leave my meeting with Dr X clear, at least, on how the system works. If you do not admit you are ill, you are not sane enough to be considered recovering. If you wish to be let out, you have to admit that some part of you is ill. Therefore, you must take pills. Rather than prescribing pills, which would at least have seemed reassuring – and would have made Dr X wholly responsible for the choice of medication – he told me to select one of three. Whatever the pills do to me will be the consequence of my choice, except that there is no choice.

It is not scientific. A doctor opens a cupboard full of medicines and says, 'Choose!' But it is honest: Dr X has no more idea than I do which one is the best for me. We could pick at random. I might as well pick at random. There is no mention of any alternative treatment, no mention of talking therapy, of psychotherapy, cognitive behavioural therapy or any kind of non-medical prescribing.

I say I will think about the pills and get back to them.

In the evening I sing 'Happy Birthday' to my boy down the phone.

Everyone says he is fine, fine, of course.

'Thanks, Dad,' he says, so dutifully. It scalds me to think of him, of what I have done to him and to all of us. I feel desperately, horribly unworthy of him. Nothing can be the same after this, I vow. It must be, can only be, better.

The queue for meds forms after supper. I am called to the dispensary.

'You're down for quetiapine,' they say.

'It's a mistake. I reported a bad reaction to it. I am not supposed to take anything until I've chosen one of these long-term pills.'

'Hmm. It's on your chart. Dr X has put you down for it.'

'But it's a mistake!'

'You can refuse to take it.'

I consider. I can't have 'refused medication' on my record if I want to get out of here. I take the pill. It makes me sick and feverish, bringing a horrible broken night of nausea, sweating and semi-consciousness.

CHAPTER 17

Day 5

A glorious sharp day breaks, cloudless. The staff squeal and goose each other with cold hands at changeover. I get up at half past seven and stare out. There is ice on the car park. Two high-vis men warm up their van. I see about eight outsiders a day, I reckon, from the various windows around the ward. The views are:

1) Sky from the foredeck yard. The yard is forty paces around, edged with lavender bushes, pleasant but so small, and overlooked from the corridor, the office and the canteen.

2) Sky from the main-deck yard. This space is twenty metres by ten and contains an array of benches; the office and various rooms look in on it. I like it less but it offers a lot of sky, and in one place, looking up over the roofs, the twigs of a treetop.

3) Portakabins, car park, low hedge, commuter car run – all from my bedroom window. In times of extreme stress (and remember, you must not show extreme stress except in a natural and understandable way) I rest my head against the cold grille that covers the window and breathe. That worked as well as smoking until dreadful Tuesday night, when the meeting in which I had placed all my hopes was cancelled.

4) The world, from the corridor windowsill, my favourite place, which is where I am now. A beeping truck reverses past my high-vis men, who are having an in-van breakfast. There is a low school-like roof behind the hedge at the edge of the car park, and then, on the skyline, a distant ridge of trees.

Stephen comes to join me at the window, pulling his hair into a ponytail. He is on ebullient form, his bright blue eyes fixed on mine.

'I love those trees over there,' I say. 'It's our one view.'

'Woolley Edge!' Stephen cries. 'You can see seven counties from up there – Humberside, Yorkshire, Leicestershire, Lancashire – and that's Wakefield cathedral! The tallest spire in England!'

'I don't believe it!'

(It turns out it is the tallest spire in Yorkshire, but Yorkshire is our England now. The rest of the country might as well be the distant, semi-imaginary globe.)

Stephen plays me music, grabs my paper and pen, draws coal seams, maps and genealogies. He is on aripiprazole today – a route I may follow tomorrow.

The fifth view is from the north-east TV room, where the Big Man likes to lie, eyes closed, listening to Smooth Radio. The Big Man has a hard, massive face. He wears a woolly hat and jacket always, as though he is about to do a bank job. He and the Sidekick Boy are always together and give the definite impression of having been in prison. They treat the ward and the rest of us with a permanent, watchful hostility. I don't think it's their fault. They are bored and probably as frightened as the rest of us.

Anyway, some wonderful person has picked holes in the opaque plastic that covers the window in this TV room. It is hard to express the happiness I feel at finding these silly little holes. Another entire view! Actually, all you can see

is a lodge with a conservatory, a lawn and a sign warning
of CCTV, but it was a new vista, a new world, when I
found it.

As Stephen and I watch the sun come up, a magpie
appears, glossy and plumped with winter light. Birds are
saviours, glimpsed from in here. Reality belongs to them as
much as it does to us. Their reality is the rushing cold of
the high air and the earth below unspooling. The towns and
roads that hold us are only knots and veins to a bird, dull
clots between fields and woods and hills of the rich wide
world. Compared to the great sea of being that they perceive,
our little days are islands, specks. There were seagulls
overhead yesterday, when I was very upset, having talked to
Dad. There was a blackbird singing this morning in the icy
dark. There were three crows last night at sunset. And this
morning, planes.

At 10.30 I am allowed to go under escort to the gym. John,
our laughing sports therapist, and Jack – bespectacled and
kind, a veteran of eight years here – take me, James, young
Adam and Jason to play badminton. On the way there I see
the world for the first time since Saturday. Oh, the unbelievable joy of it! Hedges, blue tits, goldfinches, all that *sky*. I
walk as slowly as possible, trying to drink it all in.

We pass through car parks and air and horizontal views.
Here are trees and treetops and buildings. Here are signs
and people walking; here are women in offices working. We
pass a sculpture, a mental health museum (shut) and a high-
security unit – it only takes a few minutes to get to the gym
building but we walk through a universe.

'Ian Huntley and the Yorkshire Ripper!' Jason says
proudly, nodding at the high-security unit. The hospital
suddenly seems a huge, normal world dedicated to every kind
of infirmity. I had no idea what a small part of it my ward
is: there are corridors I don't remember, wards and wings, a
broken vape-vending machine.

It is a soaring freezing day, the kind that puts a bounce in you. Jack and John do not seem to be monitoring us so much as looking forward to the session. In the sports hall they set out a net and join in. There seems to be a latent question: can we play and keep score in a badminton game like rational actors?

We sure can. We love it. I remember the sweeping, thwacking glee of hitting a shuttlecock. By turns, depending on the fall of the little flighted cone, we are triumphant, we are focused, we are delighted, we are rueful. We are free, for a little time, of all other thought.

Next we play a complicated game involving a football, something to do with assists and numbers of bounces. The gym is cut with sunlight. There are jokes; there is real laughter. It is OK to spring up and down. I feel as though all my muscles have been squashed in boxes. Now they all come bounding out.

'Why didn't you 'ead it to me?' Jason roars. All five of them are seriously good at football.

'I think it's a trust issue?' I manage.

John laughs. Someone makes a joke about broken noses.

'No offence, but give me real injuries any day!' I cry.

It is the most joyful session. They find it very funny that I simply cannot grasp the rules of the football game. You are supposed to not want to be in goal but I like goal – you forget everything but the bounce and bound of the ball; to be able to snap and slap and kick at it is such relief. James is ace, a natural sportsman, so tolerant and controlled, managing not to smash the ball into rocket flight.

We stride back across the car park different men. The happiness drains as we near the ward, but it feels as though we have been given a glimpse of who we really are.

In the afternoon I have another meeting with Dr X, splendid in his perfect shirt, suit and watch. He graciously apologises for the mis-prescription of quetiapine.

The occupational therapist blushes and looks awkward when she realises I am hoping for a home visit at the weekend. I have misinterpreted what she said about needing evidence of a home to go to. Such evidence is necessary for release but not sufficient. In here, you cling so hard to hope that you create it. Then someone has to dash it, and you want to break and hide in your room.

I present my case rationally. Dr X counters. If you don't take the pills the tribunal will order twenty-eight days. Take the pills, reassure your family (Rebecca) and we will see about making you a voluntary patient, Section 17, which will allow you to come and go, and visit home, and see your boy.

His insistence is absolute. If I want to get out, I need to take a pill. I settle on aripiprazole, as the sheets seem to indicate it is the quickest to act and the easiest to come off. But I terribly do not want to take it. The whole thing unrolls like an execution.

There is something like respect in his eyes as he adds, as if in consolation, 'If you don't like it you can always stop. It's your life. Do what you want.'

This, after pointing out that should I have another break-down I will not be able rely on being put on Section 2 (twenty-eight days) again. It will be Section 3, which is up to six months inside, renewable. I could not survive it. They are making me feel that there is something systemically at fault with me and that without pills I will get worse and have to spend my life in here. They appear to believe this so firmly that they do not seem to listen to what I am telling them.

I keep telling them that I have never had depression without a high period first. I keep telling them I have never had a high without cannabis use, and that I believe the doctor in France was right – cyclothymia, with cannabis psychosis. I don't believe Dr X knows anything about cyclothymia. He waves it away.

'All these words are bipolar,' he says.

He is so carefully generous and flattering, Dr X. He talks about my being high achieving, about being a good father, about the this and the that. And the girls, the young staff workers, are willing me on and rooting for me. They are excited and happy when I agree. I like them so much, and yet all I feel is betrayal and fury and grief. As I leave Dr X, they are waiting with the pill and the water to wash it down.

Back in my room I break into sobs. I feel they have beaten me. I took the pill with a smile and a joke for the staff. I am proud of that but I can't stop crying. Why does it matter? How stupid to cry so much, and how disgusting is this self-pity. There is a metal taste in my mouth.

I think I know where the sobbing comes from. I feel that by taking the pill I am murdering my muse. And I thought taking the pill was brave but now I realise it was cowardly. The courage of my convictions would have taken me to the tribunal, daring Dr X to blink. (They obviously don't want the tribunal: the time, the cost, the risk of their judgement being overturned, the necessity of providing every scrap of the mound of paperwork my case must have generated.)

Dr X was adamant they would not have blinked. 'The tribunal always take the cautious path,' he said.

I have taken five milligrams today. I will take ten milligrams tomorrow and ten daily thereafter. The tribunal or Dr X will make me voluntary. I will be out of here in a week, hopefully. Perhaps the pill will delete my memories. Perhaps I hope it will. This morning Stephen was roaring and crying that aripiprazole was making him ill; he could feel it, he wailed.

'It can barely have touched the sides,' the deputy ward manager said, dismissing him.

Forty-five minutes after I take the pill I feel as though something has taken sick inside me. The pill induces a ringing, numbed feeling, as though I am wearing a too-tight hat made of felt, which presses hard on my temples, dimming my vision. I can actually feel part of my mind going to sleep.

It gets dark outside. I stay in my room for a long time, writing and crying.

I make it through supper with dry eyes, all lightness gone, thinking grim thoughts about chemical coshes. On the phone I speak angrily and self-pityingly with Rebecca, then without grace or courtesy to my mother. She wants to visit. I accept her request to come tomorrow, if only so that I can see more of the grounds – we are allowed out if someone accompanies us.

The pill's effects are distinctive. On the phone I cannot link thought and feeling; I come across like a teenager, inarticulate with affront. Afterwards I reply to emails very slowly. It could be fatigue but there is something else there, a lack of fluency. I keep breaking off to space-stare. (I may not have to resist the temptation to play the zombie to needle Mum as I may actually be one.) Exercise feels futile. After some pacing outside I retreat. Around the pool table my friends save me from morbid self-pity. They see I am down and their solidarity is immediate.

'Oh yeah, Stephen's on that,' James says when I tell him what they have got me taking. He talks about neural oxidation due to exhaustion. His own fall involved ADHD and huge skunk joints.

Adam says he has been trapped by his voices for years.

'Smoking weed and listening to music, I just went inside my own head,' he says. His face looks so different, suddenly, under his hat. 'I used to work in a factory, operating machines. Then I got a kick in the head and started smoking. Weed.'

Adam says his voices tell him to kill people. He forces them down but they never quite fall silent. He was an easy presence in the gym this morning, but as we left I saw his comedown from the fun of it hit him hard. He suddenly wanted nothing more to do with anyone until he approached me this evening.

'I wanted to be army or navy,' Adam said wistfully. He was so proud yesterday, unveiling his new pool cue. He

grinned like a happy child when he was complimented on
his haircut.

Everyone confides bits of their troubles and bits of their
treatments to me. I used this in the meeting with Dr X,
arguing that it was another reason why I should be freed,
worm that I am. I said it was not my job to be a counsellor
in here. But it is, of course – it is part of the writing bargain.
I am honoured really.

The ward feels claustrophobic this evening, by its own
claustrophobic standards. Outside it is properly cold; inside
the rooms are too hot. The lighting in the rooms is horrible,
a grimy yellow wash. By switching on the bathroom light,
switching the overhead off and lying at the wrong end of my
bed I can get just enough illumination to read by, and enough
shadow to soften the room. I fall asleep at half past seven in
the evening, waking two hours later after strange dreams.
They are all visions of trades and exchanges, as though in
every sleep I peddle and swap harmonies and futures with a
happy land adjacent to this one. A consistent, coherent place
it seems, always just there, behind sleep's veil. Every time I
visit, it sends me back with a conviction, a feeling about a
thing that must be done. No doubt this is just a function of
regular contact with the unconscious, but it is beguiling.

The last ward round is quiet, an African voice returning
my 'Goodnight.' I try to speak to the watchers if they wake
me, so that I don't feel like an animal observed. I turn in,
hoping I will sleep through some of the torches, and hoping
the pill's effects fall no harder than they did today. There is
the chance of gym tomorrow.

CHAPTER 18

Day 6

The click of pool balls is often the first thing you hear. The constant sound of the ward, it falls silent only in the smallest hours. I sweat to the surface, agonising over access to my boy and the powers and convictions of his mother. Rebecca controls everything now. I lie in bed thinking about her. The size of what she has gone through, thanks to me, seems too huge to comprehend, an impossible polyhedron of stress and pain. How to begin to grip it? How to hold it? She must feel safe, anyway, with me here. I feel deeply humiliated to be locked up, but that is probably wrong. This incarceration is an undeniable fact, something that cannot be argued away or hidden. There is release and relief in that. I have been very ill. Am I still ill? I don't feel it.

It's late, eightish, when I rise. The dreams drain slowly. I have been trading again, all night it seems, bargaining my way to imaginary resolutions.

The pills are not supposed to kick in for a day or two. Was the dullness I felt yesterday psychosomatic? Are there any differences between psychosomatic and actual effects? This place teaches that there are none.

After breakfast, support worker David unlocks the larger courtyard so that I can walk out my paces.

'I used to be a banker,' he says. 'I swapped banks for the NHS.'

He had a breakdown. He talks me through it with complete openness. Alcohol and drugs drove him out of London; friends nearby brought him to Wakefield. He sees cannabis as the Devil behind so much of this hell. No one I have spoken to on the ward has not been touched by it.

It is a winter day, assertively cold and concrete-grey. A single herring gull hauls herself through the air. I move to try to keep the bird in view and she veers from her course, shy.

The morning is full of conversation and confession. I spend much of it on my windowsill in the corridor. Jason is in an outgoing mood. He ducks into the space beside me, adjusting his beanie. He is tormented by his sex drive, he says.

'There's no privacy. How are you supposed to have a wank?'

Then he tells me his father tried to rape him when he was young. His eyes shift and darken as he tells it, as if each new fact revealed is a barrier to duck behind, as if he is under fire. Watching me doing emails he says, sadly, of laptops, 'The only thing I know how to do with them is nick 'em.'

Zack comes by, bobbing and glancing. Zack and I play pool like gentlemen, setting each other up. Zack has a masturbation compulsion for which he gets free porn, the others say. He is a thin, bowed figure like a goblin from the background of a Giotto.

'A Paki spat in that,' he said, last night, of my fish pie. 'You eat it, you're going to die of Aids.'

He was referring to an Asian girl who works in the kitchens. His hatred and disgust were violent. You could actually see his self-loathing rushing out, turning into insane racism right there in front of you. It was like watching snow melting under a hot tap.

Next comes Alan, sixty-something, white-haired, a former boxer who is always dressed immaculately. He bitterly regrets drugs. 'Speed and Ecstasy,' he says. 'I took too much. Messed myself up.'

Alan is married to a very glossy lady, beautifully turned out, whom he adores. Today he says proudly, 'What's a man? I sorted out the TV at home over the phone yesterday, telling her what to do.'

We talk about being brought to the ward. 'It took more than one policeman to bring me in,' he confides with shame. He changes the subject, talking about his career. His pay-off from work was not much, but with his pension and savings he and his wife are sorted, he says, and their children long gone and flourishing.

Alan and the former miner, Arthur, have similar, east Yorkshire voices, eager for comedy, full of certainty and assertion. Arthur receives a visit from his son, a huge young man. The tenderness between them is beautiful. Arthur finds it very hard to put his leg in a painless position, he says. Only once it is settled can he sleep.

We line up for our meds. I take the ten-milligram pill. There is a bright nurse there, laughing, and another more ponderous lady who looks as though she has reached her comfort level and now has her mind on other things.

Next comes gym with John. I like him a lot. We talk about ice hockey, inline hockey and the highest climbing wall in England, which is in Brighouse, of all places.

'I fell off twice,' he says. 'My forearms were on fire.'

I wish we had a climbing wall. Presumably the authorities would worry we that we would make it a DIY gallows. We move on to his upcoming holiday with his girlfriend in Calgary and Toronto.

'She's gone from "I wouldn't mind a ring" to "Where's me ring?"'

She has my sympathy. Anyone would marry John. He is compact and sparky and light on his feet, then suddenly serious as he explains the safe usage of the thirty grand's-worth of gym equipment. It all smells newly made. When we forget where we are, and that I am technically mad, we laugh easily.

I walk, jog, row, bicycle, do weights and hard pedalling, returning to the ward feeling stretched and stronger. Everyone is in the dining room.

'What's up?'

'Lockdown. There's a knife missing from breakfast so we have to search the rooms,' says David.

We sit around. I try to read. Words will not stick; Flashman makes no sense. After a while they let us out of the dining room, the knife still missing. I sleep for a few minutes and wake, no time having passed, confused.

Woozy I wander into the day room. My friend Pete is back, talking about antidepressants and wanting to end it all. 'I only feel safe in here,' he says.

A Brexit discussion breaks out. Although most of my fellows voted or supported Leave, they now wish it would go away; it scares them. People are upset because there was a meme, in a fake BBC news font, saying that Brexit had been cancelled. Everyone's spirits rose, then were dashed when they realised it was fake. Jane, a support worker with kind lines and eyes, is horribly worried about it all. Hector, the former pool hustler, gloomily relishes it.

'The NHS is stockpiling drugs . . . You need to apply for insurance now . . . You'll need visas like you did before 1973 . . .'

He manages to get peaceful Pete going. 'Do you really think people would have voted for it if they'd known the shit we're going to be in . . .?'

Off they go. It's a squirmy time in this Leave constituency. There is anger, and righteousness at being the majority – at being the winners, for the first time for a long time, if ever – and there is fear of a humiliating rematch, and there is hope that it will all go away.

'They voted for foreigners out, that's all,' says Stephen.

The truth of this lances the room's anxiety and ends the discussion. We move on to what John Thaw died of. Death, madness and the universe are constant themes here. Adam and I discuss films about Hawking, Turing and John Nash. What killed whom and how is a constant. We cover everyone's thoughts and convictions on the deaths of Morse and other Thaw characters, and discuss his valiant wife.

'Everyone dies of lack of air,' says Hector with heavy satisfaction. His wisdom is received in sudden silence, everyone feeling all at once our lack of metaphorical air.

The knife is still missing. Staff are away training so those who remain are hassled and abrupt. We have a false fire alarm. Support worker David sweetly makes time to walk me to the canteen.

'I started training as a psychotherapist. But there were too many numbers. I like people.'

We come back. He sits and watches us plough through lunch. The catering staff are the best thing about meals. Here, they alone have no official power of judgement, so we tease, flirt, confess and ask questions.

'Doesn't she have the most incredible eyes?' Stephen sighs over one young woman, everyone's pin-up. She does. She thinks me 'right posh'. The beautiful girl and Stephen fence-flirt and make us all laugh.

I am walking in the small yard when a builder appears on the roof. He looks down dubiously.

'What's the world like from there?' I call up.

'All right,' he says.

'Chuck us a rope then!'

He laughs.

After I wake from a siesta my mother arrives. I am afraid I am horrible. For her mission to the North, Mum has dressed like a tramp in her farming gear, which makes her smell like a sheep. I refuse her gifts – moisturising cream I brought back from Italy, last used on her dog's sore ears; socks, radio, fruit, sketch book, teas. I accept satsumas. I give her chocolate biscuits to see her home. My anger is terribly childish, but I feel like a child, condemned to this place. I am damned if I am going to give into it, as it were, by taking up sketching.

At nine o'clock Mum calls; she's home. I apologise for the way I behaved. She is very gracious. It is my humiliation, we both know, and my inability to overcome a mountain of embarrassment and shame at being here that makes me act like a churl.

I call Rebecca and speak to our little boy, who sounds miserable, surrounded by meaningless toys and no Daddy to build them with. Mummy is about to give him a husky pup. ('You *are* mad,' I say to Rebecca. Rebecca seems to agree in silence. Six hundred quid, ffs.) Our boy tells me something I cannot properly hear about *Star Wars* and says, 'I'm going to give the phone back,' a couple of times, listlessly. It is torture to recall it.

I write a letter to Rebecca. As long as it takes, whatever it takes.

And then the snow comes. The men write 'Mum' and 'Dad' and draw hearts in the snow on the AstroTurf. It gets dark and I walk under shining flakes. Sometimes we are all aware of being part of each other's future memories, tender, bleak or terrifying. At some level we all know it. Young Rob makes me laugh. He is the baby of the unit, a survivor of abuse and trauma, a musician who has the inevitable skunk habit. Someone calls him on his iPad.

'I'm just taking this shot,' he says, laying the caller on the pool table's cushion, facing the ceiling. He – or, I think, she hangs up.

The Big Man and his Sidekick Boy are in the day room, bored, not watching the TV. I am idly setting up the pool balls and knocking them around when I become aware that they are both watching me. The Big Man has his strange half-smile; the Sidekick Boy in his grey tracksuit has that look of leering anticipation I have seen before. He drove Stephen to tears yesterday. 'He just poisons everything, everything,' Stephen ranted. It was difficult to disagree. Now they stare at me, and know that I know. *Do something*, I think. I straighten, lay down the cue. I approach the Big Man. 'I'm sorry, I realise we haven't said hello properly. I'm Horatio,' I say and stick out my hand. The Big Man looks at me in silence. After a long moment he shakes his head. His hand does not move.

'OK, sorry,' I say. I go back to the pool table. I can feel my face flush. The Sidekick Boy grins now. I have not seen him look so enthused or interested in anything since I arrived. As steadily as I can, I set up the balls again. You don't want to back down now, I think. *Fuck them*.

The pleasure and derision emanating from the two seated figures is remarkable. I feel sick. This is the kind of thing they understand; they love it, the motherfuckers. Still, I have the cue, so if there's any nonsense I'll wrap it around the kid's head and the big bastard will never catch me. The kid whispers to the Big Man and the Big Man sneers something back. Then he says, slowly, 'I didn't shake hands because I've got a cold.'

And so I get to apologise again, and grin, and that is that.

This evening I watch Andy, whose wife comes in and twinkles bravely at us all, negotiating for an extra cigarette. He is allowed six a day. 'With a discretionary one, and one slip,' he wheedles, desperation making him articulate. He is usually silent.

'That would make nine today,' says the care worker. She is funny and firm about it, but I cannot help seeing the guard toying with the prisoner. They split the difference, negotiating over who will sweet-talk the ward manager, who is evidently impervious to bending the rules. Andy 'presents' as one of our worst cases, disarrayed hair, lost, staring eyes, inwardly tortured, silent.

'I used to be a financial adviser,' he whispers. 'Pensions. Life insurance and investments.'

There is a slightly febrile, B-team atmosphere on the ward tonight. Stephen loses his temper and claims he had the missing knife. He shouts at the staff, 'I'll shit through the eye of a needle!'

Pete says he hopes to die in his sleep. He has checked back in, scared by the outside. Young Rob has a panic attack, late, trying to get a 'PAC-tested' charging lead. The staff rather let it all go, which creates a stringy, uncontrolled feeling on the ward.

I meet Grace, a support worker from Zimbabwe. She says fuel has tripled in price at home, hence the rioting. 'You cannot live,' she says. Her voice makes me think of travelling in the Bangweulu swamps. What an astounding life I have lived.

James and I discuss the feeling we have that one life has ended and another begun. I am sure that is right. There was a before; there will be an after; this interim is a kind of dream of death, a white nothingness haunted by spectres and reflections. My sleep is full of wakings, torches and resolutions. The subconscious is on non-stop repair, I think, searching for harmony and answers.

CHAPTER 19

Day 7

I wake thinking of Verona, of taking Rebecca her lunch at school, of Anthea, our friend and colleague, watching me come in one day and bursting out, 'You're wonderful!' And I thought, actually, I can be. It is hopeless to pursue Rebecca, to plead or beg. Dignity, confidence, humour, kindness, faith and love are all in me. It is time they had their say.

Helen and Katrina are in charge this morning. It doesn't get much sharper than that.

'No side effects yet,' I say, taking my twenty-fifth milligram of aripiprazole.

'Good,' Helen says.

I am not sure if it is true. I'm sleepy-woozy now. But then I used to sleep in the mornings on my ship, the *Gerd Maersk*, when we were crossing the Pacific.

Stepping out into the smell of the day is intoxicating. You can detect the scents of wet cold grass and earth and trees beyond the walls. AstroTurf has no smell but the sky does, and the lavender, and the fumy cold vapours overhead. There is a sting in the air of Saturday morning exhaust. When I see a gull fly over I imagine I can smell the mud on its legs.

I do not make a to-do list today. The main items are the same, always. Release the fret about Rebecca and our son, and about work, money, house, future. Release them like

balloons, push them gently away. Be. Have faith in the next
ten minutes. Rebecca is coming today. She has bought a car.

The staff summon me. Rebecca is waiting in the child
visiting room. She is setting up a new ID for me on our old
Toshiba laptop. There is a wild twisting between us of love
and missing and resentment and hope and fear and humour.
We walk in the car park. We walk into dead ends, into an
acute-care garden, through car parks, me begging for a few
more steps, a few more minutes. I read out and hand over a
letter I hope will help. Help, hope, the words are interchange-
able here. Rebecca looks pale, younger. Perhaps we have lost
years and gained time. It feels that way. Rebecca talks of
being chained to me. She is adamant she wants to keep me
here for twenty-eight days. There seems to be punishment
and self-protection bound up in it. I hate the thought of
being kept here as retribution for my behaviour but I don't
blame her at all for wanting me away from her. I cry. I thank
her for coming. We both cry.

We wipe our tears. We part well and she sets off on her
errand to buy a puppy. Her sister will drive her and they
will have time to talk. I am tormented by thoughts of twenty-
eight days.

The deputy ward manager comes oiling up. It may be
coincidental, but I am sure that he knows we are especially
vulnerable in the aftermath of a visit. The coerce-to-control
mechanism is embedded in him. They want me to drop the
tribunal in exchange for becoming a voluntary patient, he
says. Rebecca floated it too; they both summoned the twenty-
eight days and Dr X as sticks to the carrot. Going ahead
with the tribunal offers me the chance of a victory, of an
assertion of recovered sanity and health, against the risk of
being locked up for longer. Becoming a voluntary patient
would get me halfway out. I say I will think about it.

The smokers are all tooting on green-tipped e-cigarettes.
I give Jason my tobacco. A new nurse turns up, Abi, an

agency worker, I think. He can make anyone except the Big
Man talk by advancing contrary, random and strong opinions. There is quite a lot of laughter today. Young Rob,
eighteen, is hilarious. 'Bolton is fucking *shit*!' 'Prince Philip
is a sick guy!'

We roar with laughter. Apart from Rob we are all scared
of speaking freely. We police ourselves, trying to say nothing
that might offend, nothing that might count against us,
nothing that might make authority hesitate. We share confi-
dences quietly, outside and away from the staff.

'What you been doing?' James asks.

'I'm writing a travel piece for a newspaper – it was a kind
of working holiday.' Unless you speak very quickly James
loses interest and cuts in. His ADHD and amphetamine, and
the need to balance both in interaction, must require a mighty
effort.

'A working holiday? In a mental hospital? That's what my
parents said to me. I said, It ain't . . .'

We talk of fear of the future. Alan says he takes four pills
plus two pills plus four pills plus one pill every day 'to forget
what I do at night'. I am not sure what he means. Terrible
thoughts? Violent dreams?

Jason says he doesn't do the future at all.

Stephen says he will be out of here any minute. I doubt it.

There is a palpable undercurrent of sexual frustration
among us. Our eyes follow the women with their keys and
power over us, and you can feel men trying not to think
things, because we like and respect them.

Now they bring in John, who is feeble and hopelessly lost.
They abandon him in one of the TV rooms. He does not
know where he is or why. Stephen and I go to find support
worker Dan, who gets things done, to help the poor man.
Dan is terrific, short and broad and quick, unafraid of regulations, quick to smile.

'It's having the confidence to disregard the rules a bit, isn't it?' I say admiringly as he unlocks this, sorts out that and whips around doing us favours.

'Yeah!' he mouths, and grins.

On the phone I speak with my boy. He is waiting for the puppy and talking about Chewbacca and some balloons and a party he went to in his lovely Yorkshire accent! He is being looked after by his granny a lot at the moment, is my impression, which makes him very lucky. He says I can come and help him finish building something – I can't pick up on it quite fast enough but it is good, thank God. I could *dance*.

When the ward quietens, late, I go to bed with Jeffrey Archer's jail diary, volume three, which is bearable mostly because it records him having lunch with Gillian Shepherd, thereby breaking his parole conditions and getting him sent back to prison.

CHAPTER 20

Day 8

I wake repeatedly through the night, plunging back into deeper sleeps, surfacing each time sweatier and more satisfied, as if I am being unrolled and drained and expunged. Through the early light I come and go; it turns into a proper lie-in. Fully awake, finally, I say aloud, 'You are in a mental hospital being held under Section 2 of the Mental Health Act.'

Saying it feels good, even uplifting. There had to be a bottom line somewhere. When I started on this quest to be become a writer, aged about fourteen, I knew I wanted to be a writer and believed that that would require experience, varied and rich and as much as possible. I do hope this is enough.

I stumble to breakfast and learn that there are not enough staff available to allow even a walk to the front door, never mind the canteen or the gym.

Hector keeps up a monologue as he supervises our breakfast: everything we are eating, he informs us, is turning to sugar/death/diabetes. It should not be as funny as it is. He is classic.

I work. The cleaners come round. Jayne and her colleague are upset about pay and management conditions. They do all the rooms, the bathrooms and the corridors. Then they dish out roast dinner.

'There! Roast beef and all the trimmings, and your room's bin cleaned for you – what more could you want?'

'I won't say it,' I return. They laugh.

We are all very restless after lunch. Stephen and James join me in the little yard and we throw James' rugby ball. James has been here since Boxing Day. Twenty-eight days of four corridors and three rooms! And this perpetual feeling of being thought-policed. You are not allowed to think that you are well because you will then say that you are well, and we all know what that means: confirmation of insanity.

The worst of it is not that the right to assert sanity is denied us in here, in this interregnum, this non-time. The real killer is the feeling that there is no way back to normality for us. There is only a treacherous chemical bridge to a facsimile of it in the future. Every time Stephen says he shouldn't be here you can practically see them throwing away his key.

Who says we cannot get better? There must be a thousand paths to recovery. No law of the universe holds that a breakdown is a one-way ticket. And yet there is only one way out of here, through a pill bottle, the contents and consequences of which seem to be as mysterious to the doctors as they are to us.

Hector comes out into the small yard. He is great, so open and confident. Like Dan, he does not seem to check what he might say against an official template before he says it.

He was two years depressed, he says, and eventually only chased out of bed by the threat of battering or sectioning by his friend. He will be fifty-two tomorrow so has spent £169 on an hotel in Harrogate – he and his wife have booked Turkish massages. I ask him what he thinks of the ward.

He speaks in a convincing and sensible way. 'I would be happy to be treated by Dr X. He's a man who works with you,' he says. He judges Dr X an effective politician, and seems to suggest that Dr X will award me voluntary status as a way of avoiding the tribunal.

'You're doing well,' he says.

'I feel completely different to the way I was when I came in. How do I seem?'

'You presented as sane after about fifty hours,' he says.

It is a happy afternoon for a while. I write. Then comes vicious, stomach-punching cabin fever. I do press-ups and sit-ups. Outside I try walking around the yard. It is not really walking so much as square-pacing, watching distant planes and the changing, fading winter light.

Out of nowhere one of the support workers intimates that I will be made voluntary and says it is too late for me to retract my appeal to the tribunal as coercion would be suspected, but the whole thing will be now be cancelled, as voluntary patients do not get tribunals.

Yet this is coercion, top to bottom – and what they want and need is consensual coercion. Just do not tell the truth. Do not assert anything. To say 'I am getting better' is too strong. 'I am ill but hopeful' is more like it. My truth is: 'I have been fine for days and fear deterioration caused by being drugged and incarcerated.' It would be spectacularly unwelcome, though it is perfectly true.

I have a sleepy head and dulled reflexes. Writing does not seem harder than usual though, which is amazing, given the lack of nicotine. Supper is terrible sandwiches with a redemptive eclair. There is an angry farce while I try to make the bloody payphone work. I get through to my boy. He sounds very well. His pup has arrived – Lupo.

Rebecca is still hoping I will be kept in, as is Dad, but both conversations are quite good, relatively. The phone is a misery: it barely works.

One of the staff has it in for me – there is a crafty jealous power thing in her eyes when she looks at me. Dr X has not scheduled a meeting with me, she says. A wave of doubt and fear comes over me. How can he offer voluntary status if we are not to meet? Perhaps he means to demonstrate integrity and lack of coercion by going ahead with the tribunal?

Over the crap sandwiches Arthur made me laugh. 'Ah could eat a scabby oss,' he said.

It gets dark as we watch Ronnie O'Sullivan play snooker against Judd Trump. As someone who has known mental suffering, Ronnie is our man. Trump steadily beats him.

James talks furiously and quickly of how they make us act, pretend, play a part. The 'normal', everyone but us, cannot be caught out, but we are the 'acting normal', therefore obviously shamming, he says.

I chew on this question constantly. Throughout our lives we are taught to 'act normal'. At one point or another all our masks must slip. I have seen all the people I know and love best in those moments, when anger or grief or hilarity seemed to draw them out of their cover, their feelings unleashed. What are we, in those moments, if not our deep, true selves? The difference in here is that my fellow patients and I were naked and exposed for longer than a few moments; we cracked up over months or weeks or days. 'I cracked up' can mean I laughed fit to burst, or I took my clothes off and crashed my car. 'I broke down' can mean I dissolved into tears and let my true feelings loose, or it can mean I went around raving about conspiracies and Kylie Minogue. 'I lost it' can mean I tumbled into laughter or fury, or it can mean I lost my grip on reality.

This is the thing I feel we are fighting in here: the idea we are only allowed to crack, break or lose it in snatches. It feels as though, having once exposed all the wiring, having once thrown it all in the air, we are not allowed to start again or pick up where we left off. We have to be ill, now, for ever.

But I needed this breakdown. I have lived lies and dissatisfactions and worries for years. I am *glad* I broke down, cracked up and lost it. Thank God, really. It was probably this or death. The words with which a breakdown is treated are all medicalised – illness, treatment, nurse, doctor, meds – but the mechanism of treatment belongs to retribution: incarceration, surveillance, behaviour monitoring, parole. For crimes against normality, we get a label and a chemical life sentence. I hate this mechanism. I refuse to believe in it.

CHAPTER 21

Day 9

I wake throughout the night in swamps of sweat. I shout at an unknown watcher who switches my overhead light on in the small hours. There are staff shortages so agency workers come in at night and are sent to do the ward round. The policy seems heavy-handed. It would not be difficult to distinguish between who needs hourly checks and who doesn't. Anyway, if we were going to kill ourselves an hour would be more than enough time to die in. We need good sleep more than anything.

There are various discussions at breakfast. Arthur talks ceaselessly about food – 'foo-wd', 'ow much he loovs it' and 'ow bad for im' it is. Sitting near him and his relish in eating, in the atmosphere of immense certainty about who he is that surrounds him, is like being near a kind, slow fire.

Stephen talks about his band, about touring and supporting. Lee Scratch Perry has invited him to a gig. Stephen's friends come to see him often. They bring a guitar and sit strumming and singing in the dining room, defying the dulled afternoons. I can see how this tears Stephen. You feel so grateful for the effort people make for you, and so humiliated that they should have to do it, that you should be here, that you should have dragged them to this place. Before I was brought in, Stephen refused to take his pills and was forcibly

injected. It must have been a terrible scene. People still talk
about it.

I am steadily arranging my room. My bag no longer stands
by the door. I have postcards and books, things I have been
sent. First, my friend Peter Florence, that magnificent man,
dispatched a package. Inside a note: 'When in doubt – the
Master' and a volume of P. G. Wodehouse short stories.
Such kindness and lightness of touch made me cry. I have
beautiful cards from Uncle Roy and Sarah and from Dad
and Anthea, his partner. I have a poem from Jonty Driver
on a card – Dylan Thomas, 'In My Craft or Sullen Art'.

My desk is rigorously set out with writing, notes, leaflets
and papers. I have no diary so have made a record of the
dates and their events. Reading is becoming less hard, helped
by an eccentric coincidence. When Doug and Ellie came they
brought in my old Vaio laptop, which cannot connect to Wi-Fi
and has few functioning keys. Buried in the files is the manuscript of Antonia Quirke's memoir about films and men,
Madame Depardieu and the Beautiful Strangers. Antonia sent
it to me years ago, when we were neighbours on boats on
Regent's Canal. I adore the book. The wonderful thing is, I
know it. In those first days here, when the mania was coming
out of me slowly, when I could not trust books to make sense
and refer to themselves alone, reading Antonia was a magical
release. It was like having a centre to the universe – words
and stories I knew and could believe.

James is going home tomorrow. He is wonderfully excited,
reeling off the names of rugby teams he is going to try out for,
telling us how good he is at it, just like me with my Bach book.

Alan never passes me writing on the windowsill without
making a joke about how I have taken over his 'winda-sill'.
Lee seems unhappy today – there are not enough takers for
gym. Jason is very down, buried in his black hoodie. Young
Rob was wild last night. He has reversed his clock. He says
he is used to working all night on his music, so come bedtime

he is up and bursting. He ran madly around the corridors, pursued by the staff. What is he supposed to do, at eighteen, stuck in here?

At eleven o'clock Dr X puts me on Section 17. I am now a 'voluntary' patient! This means I am still locked in – no going anywhere without permission or without an escort, at first – but I am on the road to the outside.

I have a meeting with a man who will be my point of contact with the Home-Based Treatment Team in Calderdale. Andrew is soft-spoken and furrow-browed. He looks at you hard, visibly trying to work you out. Two forces run through him: the need to spend time with you, to gain an under-standing of your condition, and behind that you sense an avalanche of more pressing demands, patients in worse places, the ticking, racing clock. Andrew has driven over from Calderdale to be here, and Dr X wants him back for another follow-up meeting soon.

There are plans. I will have staff-sanctioned four-hour freedoms. In a week I will be able to go home for a night on Wednesday, returning on Thursday, when Andrew will also attend the meeting. Then there will be more nights at home and more returns to the ward, etc.

My main worry now is how much or little creative, connec-tive space the pills will leave me to work in. I feel spinny-dizzy-thick but I hope this is partly nicotine withdrawal. I have cut my intake to rare toots on my plastic tube. It could be, though the pills surely have a creeping effect.

'Horatio! Vicar's 'ere!'

The Reverend Richard Coles is in the child visit room. He has come up from London, saying he has a reason to be in Wakefield today. Everyone is in a bit of a tizz – since he was on *Strictly Come Dancing* he has become famous again: he was a pop star when he was young, and is a well-known broadcaster now. We are going into town.

'Hello, dear H,' he says, and hugs me.

'Dear Colesy. How absolutely sweet you are to come.'

'Nooo . . .'

He has brought a small fortune in pouches of tobacco, Rizlas and bunches of daffodils, the first of the year. The staff take the flowers, apologising, saying they contravene health and safety regulations.

'We'll have them in the office!' they say, delighted.

Out of the hospital we walk, and down the hill, following a path which leads down into the back streets of the town, the ring road and the shopping centre.

'What brings you to Wakefield?'

'I came to see you, silly.'

We met when I started in the Radio Arts Unit at the BBC. I was entry level, doing research, which I loved, and admin – booking studios, tickets and taxis, paying expenses and fees and filling in paperwork – which I did not love. Richard was a presenter, a star rising for the second time, erudite, mischievous, rich with the power of bringing laughter and levity into any room. We formed an immediate friendship over cigarettes on the seventh-floor balcony of Broadcasting House, a smoking area with a view over the whole of central London, our forum for gossip and the secrets of our love lives, our adventures and misadventures, our hopes, triumphs, failures and indiscretions.

The pleasure of walking with him is intense. As we stroll I am gorging my eyes on the hedges, the blackbirds – everything.

'Do you remember that dinner at the Groucho? With Mo?'

'Yes!' he cries. 'When she asked us what we wanted to be!'

He was a member of the club and a friend of Mo Mowlam. The staff knew him and were professionally unimpressed by celebrity, until they met Mo.

'She's a friend of yours? She's a hero!' our waitress whispered to Richard, huge-eyed, staring helplessly.

Mo was wonderfully uninhibited, full of Chaucerian appetite and mischief.

'What's that like?' she demanded. I had ordered pheasant, I think.

'Delicious!'

'Can I try it?'

Even as I replied her hand shot out, seizing a chunk of the meat, which she devoured as if ravenous, her eyes glinting at me (I was on my best behaviour) with huge amusement.

'What do you want to do with your life, Horatio?' she asked.

'I want to be a writer.'

'And what do you want to do, Richard?'

'I really do think I want to be a priest, Mo.'

'Well fucking *do it* then!' she cried, glaring at us like two shirkers who had finally turned up for a tutorial.

'*Nothing* makes me *angrier* than people who know what they should be doing and *aren't bloody well doing it*!'

We promised her we would.

'And here we are,' I say. 'We did it.'

'And doing it in Wakefield,' Richard muses.

'Starbucks or Caffè Nero?'

In Caffè Nero a man approaches and asks for a selfie. Richard poses with him. 'You were great on *Strictly*,' the man tells Richard. 'Cheers for that!'

'Crikey!' I exclaim. 'Is it like this all the time?'

'Quite a lot,' Richard admits.

'What's it like?'

'It's fine as long as you are in the *mood*,' he says with a look over the top of his spectacles that makes me giggle.

'But the thing is, H, I used to be able to ask donors for five grand for the housing charity I work for, and now I can ask them for *fifty*.'

'Bloody hell. You'll have to keep it up then.'

We drink coffee and eat sticky buns with Wakefield drifting around us: workers from eastern Europe, mothers with babies in prams, the elderly and the unemployed. I press Richard for more news and stories of his doings.

'But I want to know about you,' he counters. 'How are Rebecca and the boys?'

He regards me with concern but apparently without worry, without judgement. I tell him they are as well as they could be, in the circumstances – Rebecca being extraordinary, holding it all together, her family rallying.

'The important thing is to get well and come back well,' he says. 'You should take full advantage of what they're offering. You're very lucky to have it. Beds like that are gold dust.'

'I know. I am lucky. But how are you, in yourself?'

'Well H, I sometimes feel I'm watching the destruction of the two institutions to which I have dedicated my life – the Church of England and the BBC . . .'

And so he puts me in the position of reassuring him, out of generosity, I suspect, rather than need, and talks lovingly of his partner David. We cover Brexit and gossip about friends and books and art and Wakefield cathedral, and what I have found in the ward: 'Every single one of us has a relationship with cannabis. It's a fucking plague.'

Our time is too soon up. I must be back early so as not to risk being back late. Out of the shopping centre, across the ring road, through the streets of small battered houses and up the long path we pace. I am drinking it all in, the small birds, the hedges, the gulls and the unfurling clouds.

'Look at us, H! Who would have thought we would come to this?' Colesy laughs, throwing an arm around my shoulder.

'You a national treasure and me in a mental hospital! Not entirely unpredictable . . .'

'Take your time and get well,' he says. 'Your family need you back. We all love you very much, you know.'

Once, on the roof of Broadcasting House, he said something I have never forgotten. With a suddenly serious look over the top of his spectacles he said, 'Take whatever you want, and pay the cost *in full*.'

Back at the ward, under the same yellow light, with the day dying down to glum greys beyond the windows, he chats to patients and staff and says his farewell.

We hug. Off he goes in the cassock and dog collar he wears so proudly, back to the town centre and the station and a series of trains to his parish and home in Finedon. For the rest of the evening people come to tell me how much they liked him, how down to earth he was, what a good friend I have there. The staff have his daffodils arranged in vases in their office. The whole ward has been given a boost, a vote of confidence, a serious reassurance, so lightly delivered. Lucky us.

CHAPTER 22

Day 10

As a voluntary patient you are not in hospital by choice so much as cooperating in your own detention, but it feels wonderful to me. If you want to go out you need first to clear it with the nurse in charge. You agree a return time. If for any reason the nurse thinks you should not go out, or if you are late back, you can be returned to section.

'So you'll be back at two and you're going to town?'

'I want to go to the Hepworth, yes.'

Everyone seems to know about the sculpture gallery but no one has had the time to go there.

I feel newly hatched-out, raw and tentative and obvious, as though everyone I pass knows I am on day release from the mental hospital. There are flights of pigeons in the park, magpies and jackdaws. The first snowdrops are out, nodding their pure white heads at the wind. The *Spectator* has been in touch, asking me to write four winter diaries for their blog. Offers have come for travel writing and I have said yes to all of them. If all goes well, I will be going to Kenya, where I hope to take Rebecca and our boy, to the coasts of Chile and Peru, and to the Maldives. A magazine wants me to review the opening of a refurbished hotel in Malton. A whole life is pouring into my diary and all I have to do is live it. To stay well enough to live it; to negotiate my treatment so that I do not end up taking pills which will stop me living it.

At the end of the lane is an Asian barber's. Very little English is spoken here. Odd bundles of wire sprout out of the walls. Loud music plays out of an old stereo. Men converse in Urdu, and two barbers have a go at me, a young man first, unconfidently, then an older, less tentatively. They set me back on the road to the Hepworth slightly less mad-looking. I am deadly scared of running out of time, of being late back. I keep calculating and recalculating the hours and the minutes.

The Hepworth gallery squats over the riverbank, approached by a metal footbridge. Over a weir the river rushes in spate. A heron picks his way through winter wreckage, placing his splayed toes with infinite care, the wind wobbling his crest quills.

A wave of uncertainty hits me in the cafeteria. Everyone else seems so sure about themselves, so assertively sane and confident. The minute you feel you stand out you do, I tell myself. *Stop it.* Look at the river, the broken branches, the leaf litter, the bent crushed reeds, the bubbling light.

Up the stairs, in the first room, everything is suddenly better. Everything is much more than better. It is a high, wide room. The end wall, mostly window, floods it with brightness. On every other side are the pictures. It feels as though something that has been caught inside me for months is released, a held breath exhaled from a core that I had forgotten I had. The calm in which the pictures exist, and their beauty, which seems to speak in a language of silences and feelings, sway over me like music. I feel like the heron, splay-footed among the river's torrents.

Slowly I place my feet around the gallery, gazing at works by John Piper, Patrick Heron, Frank Auerbach, David Bomberg, L. S. Lowry, and, most wonderfully, in an adjoining room, an early Henry Moore sketch dated 1942, *Pit Boys at Pithead.*

For the next hours no madness, no guilt, no fear and no tremulousness has any claim on me. Beyond the rooms devoted to Barbara Hepworth's life and work is another treasure, an exhibition called 'Modern Nature – British Photographs from the Hyman Collection'. Suddenly I am travelling over and through almost a century of the country's history, its real history, its children, wastelands, blocks of flats, moors, coasts, its winds and weathers, its cars and shops.

Art therapy may sound a bit woolly and hopeful, compared to the might of a pill. The very names of the pills make them sound official, effective, unarguable. Would you rather your child was treated with clozapine or sent to an art gallery? And yet, this visit to the Hepworth seems a deep and gentle restoration of who I think I am. Further into the gallery are rooms displaying Barbara Hepworth's sculptures, her works in progress, her tools and methods and processes.

'All my early memories are of forms and shapes and textures,' she told a film-maker. 'I am the form and I am the hollow, the thrust and the contour.'

Yes, I think, that is where I am now, a place of early memory in this second, all-changed life I have been granted. Of *course* – in beginning again, in beginning to work and be again, you are remembering and relearning how to be the hollow, the thrust and the contour.

Another panel talks about her childhood, and how Hepworth believed it influenced her. She writes, 'Moving through and over the West Riding landscape with my father in his car, the hills were sculptures; the roads defined the form.'

Reading this seems to set off a line of lights in me. I grew up in hills. They made me and they continue to make my work. If healing from derangement is a process of rediscovering a lost story, of picking up the broken thread of the normal, then these quiet hours in the Hepworth are extraordinarily powerful and effective. I walk back through Wakefield a slightly different person from the tentative figure who set out that morning.

Come on, writer, I scold myself. *You know how this works. It's about the world and what you can see in it. Take a look. Take a longer, slower, look. If you would know the world then see who lives here; see how they live.*

I study the Polish shops, the halal butchers, the Chinese takeaways, the tattoo and piercing parlour. Chunky Chicken. Red Chilli.

At supper time someone mentions cannabis. Suddenly voices are rising at different tables and half of us are speaking. It is the first time so many have joined in at once. We are like a pack, baying.

'It messed me up. Completely fucked me, like.'

'And me.'

'It's terrible. Mate of mine killed himself. Skunk.'

'I was smoking that much . . .

'It's the Devil,' Stephen says. 'If it wasn't for cannabis I wouldn't be here.'

'Nor would I,' I say.

A bulky, bobbing man is admitted to the ward and Carl snorts and sniffs. 'I know 'im,' he says. 'He's my dealer.'

Later, another young man is brought in. He is dishevelled and pale, his gaze sliding sideways as though his eyes refuse to fix on anything. He is incapable of speech and he moves with tottering lethargy. He is taken to one of the bedrooms, a chair is placed in the doorway and a woman sits on it, staring at him. She stays there for a long time in an evident purgatory of boredom. Later she is relieved by another guard. He sits, sighing and shifting, truculent. He stares at the dishevelled man, who turns his face to the wall.

'What's going on?' I ask the woman.

'It's the second-highest level: constant observation,' she says. 'He's high risk of self-harm.'

'What's the highest level?'

'That's arm's length,' she says.

You do not doubt that the intentions are kind but you can only imagine how it would feel to have a large and agitatedly bored man at the foot of your bed, staring at you, as you lie in plastic sheets under bright yellow light. The next day he is moved to a more secure ward.

In the following week I go to the Hepworth daily. Each time I study *Pit Boys at Pithead* by Henry Moore, a mixture of white wax crayon, watercolour, pencil and ink, depicting four Bevan Boys at a colliery. In the early 1940s teenagers were conscripted to dig coal for the war effort. Moore found his subjects at the pit where his own father had worked, in Castleford. The picture shows four boys, their heads cocked, mobile as young birds, their helmets slightly too big for them. Behind them the winding gear of the mine looks like a menacing toy. The boys are caught between a private conversation among themselves, a world only they can understand, and their awareness of the artist, the adult observer looking and listening. They remind me of us, of me and my fellow patients, the garments of the adult world not quite fitting us, the jumbled machinery of the day-to-day not quite belonging to us, asked to give an account of ourselves and unsure quite what to say.

One of the gallery attendants says it is her favourite picture. Her name is Nina; she is doing an MA in feminist and Marxist approaches to fine art at Leeds.

'I just feel so lucky to be here, to be able to work here!' she says.

We exchange a few words about the pictures, the special exhibition of photography and the different galleries she guards. We say goodbye. I am grinning. Nina is amused, and suddenly I realise why I feel happy and grateful. This is the first normal conversation I have had for months. It is the first exchange in which I was neither manic nor mad nor known to have been mad. *You do not have to be defined by this breakdown*, I think. *You are not defined by it.*

The gallery becomes my anchor. I walk different routes to it, reminding myself that it is quite normal for me to find myself on wrong-side-of-the-tracks footpaths, in odd side streets. Wandering circuitously around feels eccentric sometimes, but it always did and it is what I have always done. I visit Wakefield library and a small museum, looking at children visiting with their mothers and thinking, one day, not too far away, I will take my boy out and we will do happy, normal things like this. With longer periods of liberty I walk for hours at a time, exploring this stolid, enduring town.

Now Rebecca calls. Our dear friend Diarmaid Gallagher, a teacher who was our colleague and neighbour in Verona, is coming to stay with her and visit me, flying over from Ireland.

'As soon as he heard, he booked a flight,' she says, and the thought of this kindness makes me cry.

The three of us meet at the Hepworth. I don't want Diarmaid to see me in a mental hospital.

'Ah, H,' he says, 'How're you doing?'

He is holding back strong emotion. We hug. He is a big unit, Diarmaid, tremendously kind and funny. He got me playing Aussie rules football in Italy. He has taught all over the world – wherever he goes he uses sport to create groups of friends. We have never spent more than a few minutes together without laughing and mocking. He is upset and worried. It is strange to see a face that laughs so naturally so strained. Rebecca looks drawn, beautiful and tense, though relieved by Diarmaid's presence.

We talk. We eat. I am out of sync with them, somehow. Not meeting in the hospital was a good thing, but I have brought the hospital with me. Slowly we lighten up. News of our son rescues us.

'How is he?' I ask.

'Ah I've been fighting your boy!' Diarmaid says with something of his habitual glee. 'He jumps on me and beats me up.

'Take your time H,' he says later, when Rebecca and I threaten to clash over how much medication I will need and for how long I will have to take it. 'Youse two need to take your time and work it all out. So that you don't get ill again. Do whatever it takes to get better . . .'

I keep crushing down an urge to protest: *No one is listening to me! I keep telling them it is cannabis psychosis; no one could have taken what I took, sleep as little as I slept, endure the stress of books and events and teaching and relationship breakdown and* not *had a breakdown. I am not mad – I* went *mad for good reasons, I got ill . . .*

CHAPTER 23

Discharge

Day 19. I am going home! Well, I am going to spend my first night at home, in the flat in Hebden, and then I am coming back tomorrow, but this is the step, the moment, the break I have been waiting for. There will be no stopping me now. I will cooperate, of course, and take the pills, since that is what it takes, and meet whoever they want me to meet and do whatever they tell me to do, and I will come back as often as they want me to but *no way* will they ever hold me again. Whatever they say, I am in no doubt at all about what I need to do. No cannabis and be careful with drink and get lots of sleep and take exercise – and be careful. Try to do less. Pay more attention to those around me. And try not to be frightened by the language, the labels or the narrative. Hold fast to your truth.

Anyway, today I am going home. Flashing up from London on the Intercity from King's Cross, Chris is coming to help. When I met him first we were seventeen and both trying to get into sixth-form college. It was a group interview. There were six of us, and Chris informed us that only 1.5 of us would be successful, statistically. In fact, five of us were accepted. I have treated most of his pronouncements with scepticism ever since, which is ironic as Chris is generally extremely well informed. His last job had him travelling the world promulgating Linux-based software, fighting the global dominance of Google, Apple and Microsoft. At one point he told me he was about to sue Google.

'You don't expect to win?' I exclaimed.

'Let's just say I think they will be surprised by the scale of the attack,' he returned with a look and a delighted *hoop* of his laughter. Since then he has become one of the forces behind the London Cycle Network, quit his job, moved his family to Rwanda and back, and become involved in the world of education.

'Oh, Chris!' my mother cries, whenever his name comes up, and then sighs, 'I wish he'd run the UN.'

Chris is all glint and dash and a booming voice I suspect he developed consciously. Mum loves his sudden sincerities. He can be as serious as a small schoolboy. When worried about you he is very tender and quiet. He loves hugely. A spell at the sharp end of the Territorial Army gave him his very straight back. Schooling in one of north London's rougher comprehensives, where he was frequently in fights for being too voluble, contributed to a fearlessness. After school we lived in France together, where we taught English and rode freight trains. He has a foolish, manic giggling side to him and a winning earnestness, when he is not mucking about.

He is squatting in the reception area when I emerge, dispatching something from his tablet.

'All right, H? Ready to go?'

'Oh so ready.'

At the station Chris buys us croissants and coffee. It is crystal-cold winter, bright with pale gold sun. Joy thrums through me. There is such pleasure in the sight of my shadow on the stones of the station, in the black nutty taste of coffee, in the company of other travellers, in the beautiful simplicity of ordinary things.

'I don't know England at all,' Chris says. 'I really want to get to know it.'

On the train we study the North as it passes in terraces and yards, in ridge lines of roofs and the blink of small windows, in warehouses and bridges. We take in the rained-on look of it all, the heaves of the moors and the twists and glimmers of the River Calder below. I ask Chris about his new job. He is going to be the CEO of a company which head teachers will call when they get stuck. Chris and his teams will sort them out. We reach Hebden Bridge.

'How long will it take us to walk to your flat?'

'About seven minutes.'

Hebden looks beautiful today, adorable, its streets inter-locked below the green fields and the wetly gleaming woods.

Chris surveys the small flat.

'Sorry about the smell. It's that rug. It came down from the house – the smell is the dog.'

'I think that rug should go.'

'Well . . . we'll see. OK, so you need to do a bit of work? I'll set you up with the Wi-Fi.'

Chris attacks his phone and tablet. I move from room to room, shuffling things about, facing the remains of the wreckage of my madness – the torn ceiling next to the bath-room, the ripped-out back of the cupboard under the stairs, the sickly smell of that candle I was burning, the black stains from the cinders of the burned cushion, the piles of rubbish I was hoarding in the box room – the map room I called it – the copies of my Bach book dedicated to figures like the finance minister of Nigeria . . .

'OK,' Chris calls, 'I'm done. Why don't I go to town and get some food while you start sorting this place out?'

Very soon he is back with a haul of pasta, eggs, bread, sugar snap peas, washing-up liquid, chocolate biscuits – I remember his sweet tooth and ferocious appetite.

Now we are tidying energetically. Chris is a lover of solu-tions, of results. He has decided to clean the windows, which need it. I am hauling and arranging and chucking out. Chris is washing and scrubbing. We calculate that it is twenty-six years, pretty well to the day, since we repainted the flat we rented in Saint-Étienne, in France. Chris puts on the music we listened to on repeat that day, all we had on CD – En Vogue and a compilation of covers called *Red Hot and Blue*.

He scolds me for only producing two chocolate digestives each with tea: 'Two chocolate biscuits are *never enough*,' he cries.

'Sorry, Chris. I must be mad . . .'

We go up the road to see Ellie and Doug, where Rebecca meets us. I see my boy at last, playing happily with his friend.

'Hello, Dad!'

'Hello, darling!'

We hug.

It is as simple as that.

With the morning comes Andrew from the Home-Based Treatment Team, and later Rebecca. Andrew seems pleased and reassured by what he finds. Rebecca is delighted and relieved Chris is here, and desperately upset and angry with the place I have brought us to, with all that I have done to us.

For a short while it looks as though we are going to nego-tiate our separation here and now, with Chris mediating. The moment passes. She and Chris are appalled by what they see as Andrew's too-tentative approach. I am talking about tapering off medication. Andrew is supportive, while suggesting to Rebecca she might go to a coffee group with relatives of bipolar sufferers. She is incredulous.

Chris and Rebecca want to see me on medication, strong, definite, lasting medication. They believe I need support to get there.

And now I must go back to the ward in Wakefield. Chris will come with me and take the train on to London.

I struggle to express my love and gratitude to Chris. He makes light of all his efforts. The train whisks him away, southwards, back to another life.

I walk through Wakefield again, up the hill, back to the hospital, looking at the low buildings and the high sky. I am shown to my room. I sleep easily now. I can read. Philip Pullman's *The Ruby in the Smoke*, a children's book, is exactly my level.

James is going home too. His parents come to collect him. We hug and clap each other on the arm and swap numbers. Stephen lends me John Steinbeck's *Travels With Charley*, about the writer's road trips with his dog.

I no longer feel constrained by the ward. All the same rules and pressures and timetables apply but none of it has any hold over me anymore. I am on top of the bills, my admin and my diary – the dullest, sturdiest pit-props of sanity. There is another trip home, and another return, and a meeting with Dr X.

Dr X is careful but insistent. 'Your presentation – a psychotic episode, your longitudinal history – if it happens again all this will have to be taken into account. If you have refused medication and you are placed on section again then obviously Section 3 might be appropriate. Cyclothymia, depressive and manic episodes – these are all terms for bipolar.'

His solution is simple. Aripiprazole for one or two years, lithium longer term.

'Right,' I say. 'Thank you,' I say.

I will meet an NHS psychiatrist, and he or she will help me make the right decision about medication.

'Right, I say. 'Thank you. I look forward to meeting the psychiatrist, of course.'

We both know what he or she will say: lithium.

Never, never, *never*.

Lithium inhibits the functioning of the nervous system. Common side effects include reduced reaction times, impaired memory, drowsiness, lethargy, slowed thinking and reduced creativity – 'cognitive dulling' in the parlance. It also causes long-term and irreversible liver damage and dozens of other side effects, but the idea of taking something that will harm my abilities to think and feel scares me more than the prospect of the damage it would do to my body.

At this point my objections to lithium, to bipolar, to the labelling and the chemical conveyor belt which seems to await me are all instinctive. I simply do not trust the system behind the doctor who faces me across the room. I do not understand how being offered a random choice of three pills could possibly represent a medical solution to a medical problem, especially as the ways in which the pills are supposed to work are mysterious. There is not something broken that they can fix: the NHS information sheets are frank about this, admitting that no one knows why or precisely how lithium or aripiprazole work.

I am sure Dr X has my best interests at heart, or at least my best short-term interests. If he believes I am likely to have another manic episode if I do nothing, then prescribing drugs like aripiprazole is the best thing he can do to safeguard my family and me. But he does not know me. He has not listened to what I have told him about how mania happens to me. Like depression – a sign that your life is making you unhappy and a prompt to change it – my mania seems to me perfectly explicable and overwhelmingly environmental.

At the end of our discussion Dr X seems to accept that there is a chink of uncertainty between what he is saying and what might actually be the case. After he fails to persuade me to have a massive injection of aripiprazole, which would remove the necessity of taking the pills, he says with a shrug, 'It's your life. If you want to stop taking the pills, stop taking them. There is no need for you to come back here again,' he says. 'Call on Monday; we can discharge you by telephone.'

On Monday 4 February, twenty-three days after I was detained, I am officially released from Section 17 and discharged, returning to the community. It is as simple as a telephone call and a filled-in form. Release comes with a care plan. I agree to take aripiprazole; I am to be visited by Andrew from the Home-Based Treatment Team; I am happy for Rebecca to be involved in my treatment as a point of contact for Andrew. I have made my objections to the drug clear, along with my wish to taper off it, should my recovery continue. All this is recorded on the care plan. I feel incredibly lucky. I believe I am free.

CHAPTER 24

Coming out

These are delicate days. In the evenings I listen to music, watch films and spend a lot of time on the Internet. I am sometimes confident that all will be well and often scared that there is no way out. I know I have been through a series of traumatic experiences and I am not over them yet. I want sex and conversation and expeditions, but the merest walk to the shops seems a shaky, cautious business. I try to do what I need to do: to eat well, relax, spend quiet time, go to bed a lot and read.

But I am out of practice at being alone in one place. The solitude I know is the solitude of travel, which comes with the turn and change of the world, the pull of the journey and the company of other travellers. To be solitary in one place is nothing like that. Daydreams and memories roam the flat. The silence seems to listen. I fill the rooms with the voices of the radio and the hopes and promises of music.

The footsteps of the lady above cross the ceiling, followed by the clicking paws of her dog. I sleep in bursts, thanks to the aripiprazole. I wake sometimes in panic thinking about my family up the road, missing them, longing for them. It is a lonely and diminishing and deserved exile. At night I think of the thousands and thousands like me, men who by our own deeds have lost our families. In other moments in the long dark hours I am easy, trusting in a future which seems both nebulous and yet somehow likely, in which we will all be together again.

Rebecca is adamant that this will not happen. I ask her twice if she wants to get back together. Twice she says we cannot. It's over. And yet . . .

Her elder son, Robin, loathes me for what I did to his mother. In his place I would hate my guts. Our son seems astonishingly resilient. Just six years old, he is suffering from our separation, from an understanding that I have upset his mother and brother, but he seems steady in himself, frank and unhidden. We all feel that Rebecca and I have a strength between us, something fundamental.

In the mornings Rebecca pauses the car outside the flat. I jump in, we say good morning and head for the station, where we put Robin on the train. We are all lifted by being together again. Robin's anger does silent battle with his tenderness. Rebecca's pride in her boys is enormous. Breakfast club, as she calls it, is very jolly. Our boy eats a bacon roll and does his reading before we take him to school. In the evenings I go up to the house to build Lego with him and have dinner with the family. Often I read him to sleep. Rebecca and I say goodnight. I walk back to town through the woods, listening out for owls. I am light on my feet because Robin, Rebecca and our son are safe and well; they love me and they know, for all my faults, that I love them.

Andrew visits, drinks coffee with me and checks on my progress. I tell him how Rebecca and I are getting on and report on my work. We are both pleased with how things are going.

Rebecca is not convinced. She is adamant that I must not come off the pills.

'Why do I want to take something I don't need?' I ask. I am in no doubt: behind the pills there is *me*. I am not mad and I am not going to go mad. Why stay on aripiprazole?

'Because you *do* need it. To alter your brain chemistry.'

She acts out of love and concern and a deep desire to take control of the situation, to ensure that no such crisis ever happens again. Taking pills – following what is known as the pharmaceutical or biomedical model – offers an apparently certain and straightforward solution. There is something wrong with my brain. The pills will fix it. Where is the ambiguity? What is the problem with that?

I understand and sympathise. Of course I must do whatever I can to make sure it does not happen again. But just suppose there is nothing seriously wrong with my brain. Suppose I have an underlying condition which can be tipped into crisis by stresses and behaviours and substances. Suppose there is no pill to remedy the causes of the crisis, only pills that suppress their symptoms. What then?

What is the right thing to do?

I start by reading, with my prescription packet of pills on the table beside the screen. First of all, what do patients say?

The Bipolar Support Group UK on Facebook is both an extraordinary space, brimming with kindness, support and affirmation, and also a wasteland of misery and distress, a daily record of the experiences of people who are cooperating in their own treatment.

Here is someone with tremors in her hands, asking if they are a common side effect of lamotrigine and Depakote.

Here someone says she forgets what she is saying halfway through sentences. She is taking 'Abilify [aripiprazole], haloperidol, lamotrigine, duloxetine, benzhexol and a few others'.

This happens 'all the time', says one. Another agrees, putting it down to quetiapine. Another who is experiencing memory loss says her doctor has told her it is caused by her medication. Yet another says it distresses her that her memory fails when talking to her daughter, which frustrates the daughter.

Another thread asking, 'What meds are you on?' generates extraordinary responses.

'Lithium, quetiapine, Valdoxan and lamotrigine for bipolar plus levothyroxine for lithium side effects,' says one.

'Olanzapine, venlafaxine, mirtazapine, diazepam, carbamazepine, clomipramine, etc.,' says another.

These are *daily* doses.

'Lithium 1000 milligrams, Depakote 1000 milligrams, olanzapine 15 milligrams, mirtazapine 45 milligrams, venlafaxine 300 milligrams,' says another, who adds that she is 'getting on well' with lithium, hopes she will be able to reduce some of the others, and that her psychiatrist has mentioned the possibility of reducing Depakote.

We know drugs prescribed for a whole range of conditions, from anxiety to schizophrenia, do help people in critical distress, and therefore their families, and their societies. Huge numbers of people will tell you they owe their lives to drugs.

We also know people who undergo decades or lifetimes of drug treatment can be made worse by them, spending years on expensive, endless journeys through the effects and side effects of different treatments, taking pills to counter the side effects of other kinds of pills.

Cruelly, those who are most obedient to their doctors and psychiatrists can find themselves subjected to a maddening kind of chemical pinball, as they ricochet through the effects of cocktails of prescribed drugs with no prospect of cure and no improvement in the conditions which caused the drugs to be prescribed in the first place.

What on earth should I do? Just take it? But suppose I do not need it? I definitely do not need anxiety, constipation, dizziness, lethargy, headache, insomnia, urinary incontinence, tremors, nausea, loss of balance, restlessness, stiffness, vomiting, a shuffling walk, difficulty speaking, drooling, blurred vision, sudden loss of consciousness, tardive dyskinesia (involuntary movements of the face, tongue, mouth and limbs) or akathisia (the inability to stay still), the last two of which are symptoms of irreversible brain damage, and all of which are consequences of taking aripiprazole.

I long for someone to talk to, for someone to say, there is a middle way. I sense that there *must* be one. Andrew mentions an NHS psychotherapist with a sixteen-week waiting time. I am broke now, but magazine and newspaper work is coming in. No one says it, but it is clear that I should return to my private therapist, if she will have me, rather than join the queue.

There is no straight way back. I am better, that is sure, but I have only vague ideas about healing. I have sex. One night, in a childish rebuke to aripiprazole, my 'long-term mood-stabiliser' as I call it, I smoke dope. Stoned and drunk, I and others scrawl graffiti on the walls of the flat. It is possible that aripiprazole helps drive this behaviour. Some of its known side effects are identical to mania – disinhibition, hypersexuality and profligate spending. I repaint the walls, return to writing and routine. I have not smoked cannabis since.

Andrew wants to know if I would like to have the monthly injection of aripiprazole, to save having to take the pills. Not entirely disingenuously, I say no; I prefer to take them daily, to have some agency in my own care. In fact, taking aripiprazole does not give me a sense of agency or control.

Within an hour of swallowing the pill I feel nauseous and overwhelmingly tired, muffled and dopey, as though I am one step behind myself, standing back from the world. The worst of the fatigue passes after three or four hours, but the sensation of being at a swaddled remove from reality remains. Constipation, check; broken sleep, check. How many more doses can I take before the more serious effects appear?

For the rest of the days I feel slightly high on it, a jiggling, unsettled feeling which translates into my writing. The articles I publish at this time are over-blown. The winter diary for the *Spectator* is packed with adjectives and images, stuffed with ebullience. A piece on a Yorkshire hotel is a rush of celebration, more like PR than journalism. My normal pace and sense of rhythm are crowded out. There is a hurried veneer over all of the work, absent only in one piece, for Radio 4, about being sectioned. This essay ends:

'The least-sung heroes of this story, I discovered, are the friends and families of those in crisis who act. To participate in sectioning someone is hard and horrible, but it is also, indisputably, to help save and redeem a life.'

On the radio you can hear a lethargy in my voice, and the tremor of fear that coming out about being sectioned engenders, but also an absolute conviction that this is a story that must be told. I believe that being sectioned has saved me. The taboo around sectioning is potentially lethal and I want to attack it.

The urgency of this project comes home to me one morning in town. My son is feeding the ducks. A small girl joins him; the children clap and giggle and throw bits of bread as the girl's grandmother and I stand watching. We fall into conversation and she tells me that her daughter, the girl's mother, is in a terrible state.

'She tried to kill herself last week. They're staying with me, and I'm terrified she's going to try again.'

'Have you told anyone?' I ask.

She shakes her head. 'She's been to the doctor, but she told him she felt better. She's going up and down all the time . . .'

'Well,' I say, 'I was sectioned. I was in a hospital in Wakefield. I haven't been out very long. But it worked – it really worked. If you call them and say she's a danger to herself then they will look after her. I promise they will. They looked after me.'

The lady says she will think about it, but we both know she will not – as she sees it – turn her daughter in.

I must do this, I think. I must tell people that they should not hesitate to ask for help, that sectioning someone you love is the kindest, best thing you can do for them. I need to explain that sectioning is not the end. You can have a breakdown and get better.

At this point, that I can continue to get better is a deep conviction rather than a proven fact. I feel myself improving but I do not believe aripiprazole is helping. When we have finished with the ducks I take my boy home and later return to the flat. It is time for the daily pill. I pop one out of the packet. A little jewel of a thing, it is small, blue and shaped like a diamond. It was worth $7.8 billion annually to Otsuka, its Japanese manufacturers, before its patent expired in 2015. Would you trust Otsuka, which funds studies of its efficacy and is in urgent search of profits since losing the patent, to tell you the minimum effective dose?

I break the pill in half, reducing the dose to five milligrams. I do not tell anyone. I want to come off the pills, off everything. I want to see who I am in myself, undosed, unaltered.

One evening in the Trades Club I meet two Hebden friends, Jill and her son Jack. Jack runs Nelson's, a popular wine bar. Jill has been working at Lumb Bank, the writing centre founded by Ted Hughes in Heptonstall, for thirty years. She and Jack do shifts there. The spirit of the place owes much to their humour, their quick jokes, their robust kindness. Jill has seen most of the great writers of our time. I lectured there once and taught there for a week. We became friends. They seem to know all about my exploits.

'Don't you think it's strange,' I say, 'that a local writer goes mad, dances naked on the roof of someone's Land Rover and crashes his car down a hill, and nothing appears in the paper? They completely missed it!'

Jill fixes me with a very bright eye. 'Do you think that's strange, do you? How do you explain it?'

I shrug. 'The decline of local papers?'

'Do you think? Or do you think there's another explanation?'

'What – someone decided not to put it in? To keep it out? To let me off?'

Jack looks vastly amused. Jill actually twinkles. 'Someone,' she says.

I exclaim, 'By not putting it in, whoever it was saved me – my family – our boy at school. Really? Really! I can't believe it.'

'We look after our own in Hebden,' Jill says.

'We look after our own!' I cry. 'I've never thought I belonged here.'

'Well, maybe you do,' says Jill.

At that moment it crystallises in me. It takes a village to raise a child. It takes a town to help save a loon. Jill and Jack laugh as I make them promise to pass on my deepest thanks to whoever was involved in the decision to spare me and my family the scrutiny and judgement of the paper's readers. Everyone we know knows about the breakdown, of course, but Rebecca and I experience it as a solidarity, a deeply sympathetic feeling of being supported, helped and hoped for, a mode that is typical of our town.

The idea for this book takes shape at the same time. By writing it all down, I will attack the taboos around psychosis and sectioning. I will explore and celebrate the role of friends, family, strangers and the professionals who helped us. I will follow a line through the layers of treatment and authority to which I was subject, from Ben, the nurse, to his management, to their management, all the way up to the member of Parliament who represents the patients in the ward, in order to understand something of the system I am in. I will find out what choices are available to people like me after we are released from hospital, and what consequences flow from them. I will seek to discover if there are alternatives to a lifetime of pills.

PART II

CHAPTER 25

In search of healing

For fun, because a journey however earnest must be fun, and for enlightenment, I begin with Zaffar Kunial, who sees things in a particular, sidelong way. It seems auspicious to start the journey with a poet's perspective. Throughout the paranoia and madness, Zaff seemed to me to be trustworthy. I attributed secret lives and agendas to everyone except for Zaff and another writer friend, Ben Myers. I want to know how Zaff saw what happened, to discover if there was something in the way he behaved and treated me that might hold a key to his mysterious power of deflating or deflecting my madness.

We meet at the coffee shop by the ducks. Zaffar looks well, jacket elegantly dishevelled, beard and moustache somewhat trimmed, hair standing up as it does, his eyes bright with pleasure and kindness. He always makes me laugh.

First, he asks for 'a weak latte', then when it comes he produces from his pocket a pat of butter made from goat's milk.

'Have you heard of bulletproof coffee?' he asks.

He dumps the white pat into his mug.

'No!' I laugh. 'When I do that kind of thing people think I'm nuts . . . I went through a stage of putting raw eggs in pints of Guinness.'

We talk about poetry and cricket, butterflies and cities and Sylvia Plath, whose grave is on the hill above us. Zaff says he has walked there a hundred times.

'It's just the right distance for a walk. Last time it was covered in butterflies; amazing, just her grave, so many of them.'

We discuss Ted Hughes' inscription on the headstone: 'Even amid fierce flames / the golden lotus can be planted'.

It seems generous and deeply welcoming to the thousands Hughes must have known would come. We talk about the valley and the privilege of having Plath up there, above us all who live in Hebden Bridge. Zaff produces two of Philip Larkin's collections, glowing old Faber classics.

'Have you heard?' he says, frowning. 'They say so-and-so is "in the bin", or so-and-so is "cancelled". Whitman's cancelled. Racism.'

'Cancelling', he explains, is a Twitter-based movement originating in the United States, a branch of social media shaming applied to poets and public figures whose lives or work in some way offend.

'Christ!' I exclaim. 'What about Ted Hughes? That's the language of fascism!'

'They're very keen on calling people fascists. It seems to take no account of context or anything.' He starts laughing. 'I sometimes think, *Thank God I'm brown!*'

'Thank God I've got mental health issues!'

Zaff is the easiest company, funny, sympathetic, deeply kind. You could tell him anything.

'So the thing is,' I begin, 'it's as though I died. Being sectioned, the whole thing – I feel as though someone died. So I'm trying to understand it by hunting a ghost, in a way. Tracking down a dead man. Looking for eye-witnesses.'

Zaff nods. 'That makes sense. A kind of double haunting – you're looking for him, and he's sort of looking for you?'

The idea of my past self looking for me is uncomfortable, and true. In the myth of the doppelgänger, much depends on who sees whom first. If you see your double and he looks frightened, you are the real one, the other the shadow. But if you see him and you are scared . . . I am not scared of facing who I was but I am terrified of ever being him again.

'Can I ask you what I was like?'

'You kept bringing me presents! You gave me a pen. And an ashtray, which I didn't need at all. I appreciated it; I tend to have quite quiet Christmases – I thought, *At least I've got H's random presents*. One night you came with a Christmas tree. A huge Christmas tree, after Twelfth Night. I had a non-Christmas apart from your presents. One night you left a bag of clothes. It was often around midnight. Another night you left a bottle of wine.'

'I am so sorry, Zaff. Did I make any sense?'

'No, honestly it was fine. Your individual sentences made sense but sometimes they were not connected. You didn't want to talk about home – you were travelling, perhaps that's what all the travelling was about, in the car and in your mind. You refused to settle. It's that Hamlet thing – it's articulate but the mind leaps from one thing to another without the intervening sentences. Whenever I said, "How are you feeling?" you would very soon find a way to talk about literature again. You wouldn't look at what was going on with your life. I realised you'd come out to talk about something else.'

He reminds me that he had a deck of Rumi cards, like Tarot cards, and that I had thrown some of them into his fire. I remember doing it.

'When I saw you throw the cards into the fire I saw the destruction – the throwing into the fire – and I think you weren't registering what you were doing. I thought you were going through something – a heightened state I didn't label it; I was ready to go with you wherever you were going. I didn't have a label for what you were experiencing. And also I'm a poet and I understand that heightened experiences are where it all comes from. It wasn't far off inspiration, sometimes.'

'I remember feeling safe with poetry,' I say. 'And wanting to be a poet – you know, poets can walk at night and commune with the dead and speak in tongues . . .'

He nods. 'It's as though you wanted that permission. You would get poetry books off the shelves. You talk about poetry better than most poets.'

'So do you feel you enter a heightened state when you're writing?'

Zaff smiles and looks suddenly impish.

'I almost have to act like I don't care. I'm around and wandering, going to cafés, and it's like the poem is at the edge of the table. Most of the time my poetry is actually the edges of things. I try not to label things . . . Poets have difficulty calling something one thing. I'm a poet of gaps and spaces. I think that's why I like butterflies. They seem almost peripheral beings that catch the edges of things. It's about the fluidity of things. Who wouldn't want to be visited by an articulate friend with a bottle of wine? You were very sunny.'

He produces his iPad, which looks as though it has been run over, words and spaces carefully laid out behind crazed glass. He asks for thoughts on three poems he is preparing for a pamphlet. They are built around cricket but they stretch far away, to childhoods, to other lives, to still places. One line runs, 'We all have lives that go on without us.'

'I got that walking along the canal,' Zaff cries. 'Ten syllables too!'

We laugh, delighted. Too soon we say goodbye and go back to our work.

I walk back to the flat ruminating. Zaffar is right. We do all have lives that go on without us. We all have deaths that did not take us, too. How absurdly lucky I am to be here, still, and to be setting out in search of the lessons my odyssey might have to teach.

It was Zaff's refusal to judge, to fear or to suspect that made him a safe confidant. *I was ready to go with you wherever you were going. I didn't have a label for what you were experiencing.*

What an interesting approach – to treat a manic high as a kind of creative state, as an experience someone goes through; to treat me on my own terms, freeing both of us from the anxiety of a label. In Zaffar's way of seeing, in his response to the world, I recognise a spirit which I believe underlies all writing, all art. It is a rejection of the familiar which masks the actual, a certainty that everything may be seen – deserves to be seen – as if for the first time. It is the conviction that creativity and creative ways of being begin with a radical openness to possibility.

My appointment with the NHS psychiatrist, Dr Y, is approaching. I am half scared and half hopeful. For all my suspicion of labels, I decide I will be frank and optimistic. I will tell him the truth and listen to what he says. I am feeling well; I am on top of things; I have love and purpose and faith. There must be a hundred ways forward from here.

CHAPTER 26

Chemical warfare

The appointment with the psychiatrist falls on a day of fragile sun between the end of winter and the start of spring. Andrew from the Home-Based Treatment Team and Rebecca will accompany me. It is thought important that your nearest relative or carer – who does not actually have to be related to you, or officially designated your carer – should come with you to a meeting like this.

Rebecca and I are getting on well. We are sharing the school run. I am often at the house with the family for meals and spending less time at the flat. Bit by bit we are coming back together.

Dr Y is a lively man in late middle age, smartly dressed in an expensive black suit. He has reviewed my case while we were waiting in the lobby. I suspect it has taken him about ten minutes, at the outside, to scan the paperwork.

Rebecca and I lean forward on our chairs in his office, hopeful and respectful, beaming expectation at him.

'How are you?' he asks.

I say I am very well.

He runs over my story in broad outline.

'And there is a family history?' he prompts.

'Yes. My father suffers from depression. My sister committed suicide in 2011.'

'And you say you go high in the autumn, and then low in the winter?'

'I have done. I feel optimistic and creative around September, and I am seasonally affective. But with vitamin D and exercise—'

Rebecca joins the conversation. Dr Y is keen to hear from her. She tells him I have had high periods and low periods since she has known me, over the last ten years.

I counter that I believe I am strongly affected by cannabis, that I have never had a high without using it, and that I trust the diagnosis I received in France – cyclothymia.

Dr Y replies that with my longitudinal history, and my family history, he is in no doubt. 'This profile is bipolar disorder,' he says.

Rebecca looks tremendously relieved. If there is a diagnosis there will be a treatment. As long as I submit to it, she can stop worrying that she and the children will be dragged through the hells of living with me while I am manic or depressed. I understand. Half of me feels that if there is a pill I can take that will guarantee her peace of mind, a calm and stable home for the boys and all of us back together, then I should just take it. And yet, Dr Y is here to treat me, not her. And he is not listening.

'But I have no history of mania without cannabis,' I press. 'And I have never been depressed without getting high first.'

Dr Y is inflexible. He seems uncomfortable with this information, as though it is a distraction.

'What are the options from here?' I ask.

'I recommend lithium,' says Dr Y. 'If you take it long term there is every chance you will not relapse. If you do not take it the chances are you will experience another episode – more frequent episodes, and they will be more severe.'

I explain that I am a writer. The accounts I have read of lithium are replete with stories of users becoming numb, cut off, cocooned within themselves, feeling separated from the world.

Dr Y listens to these worries but we can all sense his impatience. The fifteen-minute slot is ending. He has made his diagnosis and recommended treatment. What more is there to discuss?

'I would like a second opinion,' I say.

Dr Y looks baffled.

'I have over thirty years' experience,' he says.

I like Dr Y as a person, from what I can tell of him. In no way do I wish to impugn his skill or his motives. But this is my life and my career: why should I not have a second opinion?

It becomes rapidly clear that people in my position do not ask for second opinions. Andrew looks troubled and uncomfortable. Dr Y does not know where I would go to find another opinion.

'But supposing I am right,' I plead. 'Supposing it really is cannabis psychosis. What would you recommend I do then?'

Dr Y shrugs impatiently.

'Well if you don't use it for two or three years and nothing happens then . . .'

I press the point: I have never felt high or exhibited signs of hypomania without cannabis use. I wrote a book about it, I tell him. I have evidence that cannabis causes my mania.

Dr Y, with support from Rebecca, is firm. He thinks it is more likely that I start to go high and then use the cannabis to self-medicate. He informs me that that is the case.

There is more I should say but I can see he will not change his mind. In 2007 I published a memoir, *Truant*, which reported the effects of cannabis use on me and a wide circle of friends, acquaintances and interviewees. All of us had been knocked sideways by cannabis in ways which were more serious than society at the time seemed to understand. A tenuous link between cannabis use and schizophrenia was all that researchers would admit, while I found abundant anecdotal evidence of depression, mania and psychosis inspired by cannabis. I found that smoking propelled me to hypomanic highs and that when I stopped I came down, felt blue, sometimes black, then levelled out. I concluded the book by saying I would never be safe around it and vowing to avoid it. I am sitting in Dr Y's office, I am quite sure, because I broke that vow.

As I talk to Dr Y and Rebecca I am entirely sane. I have capacity. I have insight. I am not experiencing delusions or flights of ideas. As the *Oxford Dictionary of English* defines 'sane', I am 'of sound mind'. Dr Y and I are disagreeing over the second part of the dictionary's definition: 'not mad or mentally ill'. He thinks I must be, because I have been in the past. I am sure I am not.

How many thousands of us have sat in rooms like this, being treated like this? Here is Dr Y in his smart suit, with his qualifications, his experience, his generous salary (you can start on £105,000 in our area as a consultant psychiatrist) and his power. And here is me, recently released from a mental hospital, protesting my sanity.

Even without Dr Y's power, I am outnumbered. Rebecca is in the position of hundreds of thousands of those who love and care for people who have been or are mentally ill. As she understands it, I have a chemical imbalance in my brain. Dr Y's pills will remedy it. I cannot fight them both.

We agree I will stay on aripiprazole for now. When I ask Dr Y what it does – for I am still innocent of psychiatry's ignorance as to how their drugs actually work – he says briskly, 'It brings you down if you go high and it brings you up if you go low.'

I am confused. How, by adding a set of chemicals to my system, could both a deficit and an excess be remedied?

We leave the surgery. Rebecca is reassured by the diagnosis but uneasy that I am resisting it. Andrew is worried for me. I am reeling.

I have a few certainties: I am not going to take lithium; I will get a second opinion; I cannot contemplate the choice which is forming on the horizon like a pall: take the pills and keep your family, or resist, keep yourself and your abilities intact, and lose the people you love.

I write to Dr Ranjan Basu, consultant psychiatrist and clinical lead for South West Yorkshire Partnership NHS Foundation Trust, Dr Y's superior. I explain the situation and humbly request a meeting, saying I hope to explore all possible treatment options.

Dr Basu responds within the hour, via his secretary, saying he cannot spare the time to meet, now or at any foreseeable point in the future, and recommending I talk to Dr Y again.

The policy on second opinions, in the case of questions around a life-changing, life-defining treatment like long-term lithium, is, go back to the first opinion and do what you are told.

I know I will never agree to take lithium and I am resolved to come off aripiprazole as soon as possible. Rebecca is adamant I should not come off – the pills, to her, are a form of guarantee upon which the family's safety depends.

Dr Y is more sanguine. 'I don't want anyone to be taking aripiprazole who doesn't need to take it,' he says, in our second meeting.

The social worker, Andrew, going on what he can see in front of him – someone well, who wants to come off anti-psychotics – seems in favour of tapering off the dose.

At the end of the second meeting we compromise. I will take a daily five-milligram tablet of aripiprazole, principally, in my view, for the sake of Rebecca's state of mind, and we will have a month's supply of ten-milligram pills for use should I exhibit signs of mania.

Secretly, having already halved my dose, I have an alternative plan. I will come off aripiprazole and hoard a stash of five-milligram pills as well as the emergency packets of tens. If I start going high I will take fives, and if necessary tens, whatever stability requires. I will find out if it is true that without cannabis I am fine. If I am wrong, and I start to come up, then I have a safety net.

CHAPTER 27

Spring

It is now late March, a month after my release from hospital. From reading about the side effects of aripiprazole and lithium and studying the testimonies of patients, academics, psychotherapists, psychiatrists and journalists who are hostile to psychiatry's present configuration, caricatured as 'a pill for every ill', it is easy to discern a serious division between psychotherapy and psychiatry about how mental distress should be understood and treated. Psychiatry views the causes of disorders as multiple and complex, almost beyond reckoning. It addresses their consequences with medication. Psychotherapy seeks to address and treat those complicated causes, accusing psychiatry of merely medicating and masking the symptoms.

At this stage my aversion to aripiprazole still remains primarily based on instinct (I do not want to take something brain-altering if my brain does not need it) and on curiosity: what will happen if I come off this pill?

I decide to find out. A magazine has asked me to write about a cruise up the west coast of South America, from Valparaiso in Chile to Lima in Peru. Ten days of being pampered at sea, with shore visits suitable for pensioners, must be the ideal circumstances in which to come off an antipsychotic. I quit the pills.

From the ship I write to Rebecca and our son:

We flew over the Atlantic Ocean for ages, the moon shining down, the clouds glowing white and still, and the ocean dark and peaceful below them. When the light came we had crossed Brazil and now the Andes were breaking through the mist below us, red mountains like Morocco, the very highest peaks with snow on them. And much of Chile is mountain, parched and dry like the Atlas, nothing growing for miles until you reach the coast. The Pacific Ocean was hidden under white cloud. We landed at the edge of it. Everyone walks very slowly in Chile . . .

Rebecca and our boy write back. We begin the most wonderful correspondence, brimming with love and hope. She writes:

It was so lovely to read your email today and to feel involved with you again. I do love you so much. Robin made me cry today when he said that it sounded like the Horatio he first met.

And, we did have a proper adventure driving over the moors in the pouring rain trying to get home after swimming, praying that the new flood defences would not break! There were manhole covers burbling and spurting out water and old men in galoshes trying to clear drains and throwing down sandbags. I fear there will be a lot lost, but not to the extent that it was last time.

The dogs are still refusing to go out, they are still sat under the table and are growling at each other over a bone, but not fighting, as that would involve leaving their sanctuary under the table. We are going to eat supper now and then get in bed and listen to the storm and read 'The King Must Die'.

Email me, lots, love you x x x

We write every day. A discussion arises about different forms of love. It emerges that although I have heard of

agape and Eros, I am ignorant of the richest kind of love.
Rebecca writes:

> I am being observed at work tomorrow so I am off to make
> a fantastic PowerPoint on *Still I Rise*; will have to hold back
> for the first session and just be very analytical – but the
> observation is only for an hour. Will then have feminist rants
> in my lessons for the next three hours. Sometimes, I just
> love my job.
>
>   Pragma, my love, is the enduring love of lasting couples
> – it is a really interesting one at the moment as it is a devel-
> opment which is experienced over time and comes through
> compromise and wishing the best for one another. It is a
> development of Eros, and in Socratic terms allows the full
> realisation of it. I will tell you all about it when you get
> back. xx

I reply:

> My love I have never even heard of pragma. For Gods' sakes,
> this is where I have been going wrong. I love it when you
> write to me. You are the most hidden open person I have
> ever known and I do love you for it. When you write I can
> see you – you, whom I love more than anything, you with
> all your bright brilliance and humour and your armour off.
> Now I will look for pragma . . . nit that I am. Sleep well
> darling. I love you x x x

Aripiprazole leaves your system quickly. The fuzziness in
my head evaporates. The ship forges through seas the colour
of whales' backs. As we manoeuvre in and out of the harbours
of Coquimbo, Iquique, Arica, Matarani and Callao, I interview
passengers, the captain and the crew. I take copious notes on
the excursions ashore. In doing what I love I feel as though
I have come back to myself, or at least that I am coming

closer to the person I hope and want to be – someone calm, productive and sane. Rebecca and I write daily. I send messages to our boy about turkey vultures that slide down lamp posts, pelicans that wink, sea lions that swear and jellyfish the size of cows.

Talking to people is wonderful fun, lit with the relief of thinking about anything but me, of thinking about the world, its travellers and their histories. They do not know I was ever mad. I am a slightly odd presence on the ship, younger and more solitary than the other passengers, and working while they are holidaying, but it is an oddity I know. I am who I was and will be, I think. I am staying off this drug.

Not long after returning I am due to travel again for work, this time to northern Kenya, to a desert lake, Turkana. Rebecca and our little boy are going to come with me. I tell Rebecca I plan to come off the pills. I am hoping she will understand, and that when I tell her – months hence, when I am demonstrably fine – that I came off them a little early, she will not be upset. She is horrified.

'If you stop taking it, we are *not* coming to Kenya,' she says.

I think about it. I know we need the trip – it will be an adventure, a holiday, a rare and tremendous opportunity. At the same time, I fear aripiprazole terribly. I do not trust it to do good and I am assured it will do harm.

Our boy needs his parents together, his father well and his mother unburdened by worry. I am certain that if I tell Rebecca I am off the pills and determined never to go back on them, she will insist we separate.

How do I weigh Rebecca's right not to be lied to against our child's right to two loving parents, our responsibility to provide that, if we can, and my right to decide on my own treatment?

I long for her to say, 'OK then, I will support you in this. Let's try coming off it . . .' But her intransigence is entire, and entirely understandable. She cannot contemplate any risk of me relapsing into mania or psychosis. Dr Y has given us to understand that aripiprazole is a guarantee against that.

In the end I can see only one solution. I decide to lie. I can only trust my conviction that I will stay well, that the emergency stash of pills will get me through if I am wrong. I believe that the love between Rebecca and me and our boy is worth this undoubted sin on my part.

Faced with a choice of inflicting brain damage on yourself or telling the truth and losing your family, no doubt better people than I am would not even consider lying, and opt instead for one or the other. I can only admire them.

For two weeks, on our way to Turkana and back, we live out of a Land Cruiser, sleeping on stretcher beds in the open. There are two other small boys on the trip, who become our son's heroes. We travel hard hours into vastness, to the desert lake and on to Marsabit, a mountain above the plains, and on to the Laikipia plateau. Our nights are gusted by the hot winds of the Somali border. We walk through petrified forests. We watch elephant, giraffe and antelope. We remember how well we travel together.

'He's a different boy since you went to Kenya!' says his teacher after our return. And he is – a bubbling, bouncing boy of a hundred plans and a thousand questions.

Rebecca glows with the sun and the journey, as though something in her that was wound tight has uncoiled.

Back in Yorkshire, with the late spring singing through the valleys around Hebden, it is time to pick up the quest again. I need to find out whether there is actually something biologically wrong with me, something which science can identify and remedy. I want to know what the phrase 'the mental health crisis' in Britain refers to, and I am determined to find and explore the most hopeful avenues for the future of treatment.

I need an expert. I want a practising psychiatrist, someone who can explain current thinking and turn an open gaze on the future. A friend, a senior project manager at Guy's and St Thomas' Foundation Trust in London, identifies the very man.

CHAPTER 28

Radical psychiatry

I meet Dr Peter Macrae in King's Cross. Peter is a consultant psychiatrist who works in east London. He seems young for his position. He laughs when I mention this, saying he's been a consultant for a decade, claiming it is not hard to progress quickly in his field. Peter is very energetic for someone who has just recovered from an operation for acute appendicitis and an infection arising from surgery.

Plain in his speech, his gaze is friendly and curious behind his glasses. Bearded, wearing a sweater, tracksuit bottoms and trainers, he talks rapidly with a soft Scottish accent.

'I'm an assistant clinical director of in-patient services,' he says. 'I'm currently on secondment working on digital systems. I did a lot of work on severe psychosis – the most ill people in the country. The last two or three years I've been working with less severe cases, looking at diagnoses and screening for ADHD and the autistic spectrum. I've switched from seeing patients all day to doing a one-hour assessment, making sure there's a plan in place. It's a nice change of pace.'

We both have young children. Peter's work on digital systems, he says, allows him to see more of his.

'I'm trying to understand brain processes in mania and psychosis,' I tell him. 'I want to be able to explain to the general reader what we know about what goes on in the brain, and where we are with treatment. I want to understand how the current model is working, if it is working. For example, I have read claims that instead of investing in new treatments, the pharmaceutical industry puts its money into marketing old ones. I don't know if that's true?'

Peter nods. He looks grave.

'At the moment we're in the position where drugs that work are no longer profitable for the drug companies and are being withdrawn from the market. [When the patent on a drug lapses, the drug becomes unprofitable.] I've got people who are managing well, with no side effects, on things like piportil and clopixol, and we're having to tell them we only have supplies to last them until January.'

'What are they going to do then?'

'Well it's person by person. How likely is it that they still need it at this dose? Can they take something else? We'll try the next drug. If their life is still chaotic, could they move to fortnightly injections instead of taking it orally daily? Can we get by on a lower dose? It needn't be a disaster, but there are indications of many instances of drugs being removed from the market not because they were ineffective, but because they were unprofitable.'

I outline my breakdown and treatment, telling Peter that I was hospitalised, and that the psychiatrist I saw told me that the breakdown and psychosis means I am bipolar. He recommended lithium. I tell Peter I don't want to take it. I do not tell him I am not taking the aripiprazole.

'I'm prescribed five milligrams of aripiprazole, which isn't supposed to be a therapeutic dose.'

Peter shifts in his seat. 'I wouldn't necessarily say that.'

'I'm convinced I'm cyclothymic and predisposed to cannabis psychosis. If I'd never smoked it, I don't believe I'd be anywhere near this position.'

Peter looks thoughtful. 'Sounds like a fair shout,' he says quietly.

In the context of our interview there is no time to stop
and take this in, but I feel wonderfully thunderstruck. *Sounds
like a fair shout!* Finally, someone has listened.

'So, what do we know about what was happening in my
head as I started to go high?'

'Do you know about the dopamine hypothesis? It's the
main mechanism we have for explaining positive symptoms.
Positive symptoms are hearing things, seeing things, delusions – these are the cultural historical indications of these
illnesses. Positive symptoms include hallucinations and
abnormal beliefs – meaning false, unsubstantiated, inappro-
priate ones. So not the God delusion [the idea that God
exists, rather than the idea that you are God]; we're talking
significantly at odds with mainstream beliefs, possibly threatening to personal safety. Everything's on a spectrum, and
it's all mashed up in reality. A genetic history is not sufficient
to cause positive symptoms, there may be overlaps with
experiences, social causes, attachment or emotional disorders,
it can be nebulous or it can be definitive, the result of abuse.'

Peter is the most engaging speaker – quick, sure of his
ground and unfettered. He evidently knows the field well
enough to be fearless in his judgements and confident of his
insights.

'The sense of identity and self-worth may be unsupported;
they may present with stress, substance abuse, lack of sleep
– many things,' Peter continues. 'The dopamine hypothesis
gives one main positive factor: an excess of dopamine in the
brain pathways, specifically in the main mesolimbic pathway.'

This seems to make chemical sense of my experience. The
pleasure, excitement and challenge of touring my books, of
teaching, of beating the teeming demands of my diary, of
non-stop travel, plus alcohol and cannabis, would have
flooded my mesolimbic pathway – also known as the reward
pathway – with dopamine. By the time I reached the airport
for our flight to Innsbruck, with the prospect of the snow

and the mountains ahead, it would be reasonable to suppose my serotonin and dopamine levels were boosted well out of their normal range.

'Old-school antipsychotics worked by blocking the D2 receptor. [Dopamine receptor 2 is found on neurons throughout the central nervous system. Nerve impulses in the brain travel across junctions called synapses. Receptors on either side of the synapse release and receive chemical messages. There are in fact two kinds of receptor, pre-synaptic, before the junction, which regulate the release of dopamine, and post-synaptic, after the junction, upon which the dopamine acts. The D2 referred to here is the post-synaptic. Researchers now worry that antipsychotics also block the pre-synaptic D2 'autoregulator', which has the effect of increasing dopamine production, which explains why relapses can be so severe when antipsychotics are withdrawn.] Both generations of antipsychotics block it. The first generation have a high affinity to the D2 receptor so they block it hard; the second-generation drugs also block serotonin and histamine receptors. They are essentially mood stabilisers. It's quite hypothetical how lithium actually works. You know it was discovered as a side effect for treating gout?

'We can look at the ion channels and membranes, at how intra-cellular membranes change, we can look at the details of changes and the effect lithium has, but in terms of the web-like interconnectedness of how lithium actually works, we don't have that level of understanding.

'So we have the dopamine hypothesis and then there's the monoamine hypothesis, which is about moods. They are affected by serotonin, noradrenaline and dopamine. Antidepressants work on one or more of these three. So fluoxatine and citalopram are selective serotonin reuptake inhibitors – they bulk up transmission of serotonin, keeping serotonin near the nerve junction. Then you have SNRIs, selective noradrenaline reuptake inhibitors, like venlafaxine . . .'

Peter outlines two more hypotheses, histamine supplementation (histamine is a powerful regulator of the hypothalamus, which controls hormone release) and the glutamate GABA hypothesis. Glutamate and gamma-aminobutyric acid (GABA) are neurotransmitters. Sodium valporate, which I was offered, increases the presence of GABA, helping both depression and elevated moods. Too much glutamate in the brain is thought to cause anxiety and insomnia; too little and your brain fogs, you think less effectively and your memory is impaired.

Simply put, antipsychotic drugs act on receptors, either blocking or increasing the transmission of dopamine, histamine, serotonin or glutamate with the aim of regulating mood.

'The point is to bolster the systems that influence equilibrium,' Peter says.

To me it sounds, if not straightforward, then solvable. Identify which neurotransmitter, from dopamine to glutamate, is out of line, and prescribe the appropriate balancing pill. But Peter shakes his head.

'We have no useful tests. Researchers in a lab may be able to see chemical interactions. There is evidence for brain changes in mania and psychosis, but the variation is not far enough from normal variation to be useful. There is some grey-matter loss in psychosis. But we have no blood tests that can help us – all our treatment is based on presentation. We could say, these systems are not functioning, these systems are abnormal, we can identify points of dysfunction – but we can't look into the brain.'

We can't look into *your* brain. We have no scan which can measure and assess all the different processes taking place in your brain; nothing that will produce a useful, comprehensive conclusion. The brain's systems and processes are too various, too complex and too intertwined for any scan to give a definitive answer as to what is happening in the brain of someone in the throes of psychosis, for example. As Peter says, all we have established is that there is evidence for brain changes in psychosis, but, apart from grey-matter loss, other variations are not statistically significant. (While white matter is located deep in the brain's core, grey matter covers its surface and contains most of the neuronal cells, responsible for muscle control, sensory perception, memory and emotions, among other things. Many of the side effects of psychiatric drugs are symptoms of changes in volumes of grey and white matter.) Researchers have studied brains living and dead, brains pre-medication, post-medication and never-medicated. They have scanned brains in different stages of mania, psychosis, depression and schizophrenia. Instead of bolstering the dopamine and similar hypotheses, this accumulated research has led many psychiatrists and neurobiologists to conclude that mental distress does not start with chemical imbalances in the brain.

Schizophrenia was long held to be a result of a malfunctioning dopamine system. Molecular neuropharmacology now confirms that there is no evidence for this. Excessive dopamine synthesis and signalling is a feature of psychosis and schizophrenia, and dopamine abnormalities may be present pre-psychosis, but although these changes are clearly symptomatic, there is no evidence that they are causal.

As for depression, no chemical imbalance has been found in an unmedicated brain. In psychosis, 'evidence suggests that psychosis is the result of a network dysfunction that includes a variety of brain regions (and multiple neurotransmitter-specific pathways), of which impairment at any level could precipitate psychotic symptoms', as the journal *Translational Psychiatry* put it.

While the serotonin, dopamine, monoamine and histhamine hypotheses remain unproven, the long association between psychiatry and the idea that psychiatric disorders are caused by chemical imbalances in the brain now makes many psychiatrists deeply uncomfortable. Professor Ronald Pies, editor in chief emeritus of the *Psychiatric Times*, wrote recently in that journal: 'With 20–20 hindsight, the imbalance claim has proved inaccurate and simplistic . . . Even today, we simply do not have the sophisticated technology to verify or falsify, in real time, putative neurotransmitter "imbalances" in the human brain.'

I think back to the rising tide of mania. As Austrian Airways' morning flight from Manchester lined up on the runway at Innsbruck, my brain was a tumult of boosted and depressed transmitters, if only in terms of my drug and alcohol intake in the preceding days and my feelings in the moment. Cannabis at low doses increases serotonin; at high doses it flattens it. So, ironically, the very small joints I was smoking, in an attempt to limit its effect, were making me higher than if I had rammed them with hash.

Alcohol increases dopamine release while damaging the dopaminergic system – the system that produces dopamine. (This is why alcoholics need more and more drink to get the euphoric feelings they crave.) Add the releases and reactions in my emotions and neural pathways at the gleeful dazzle of the mountains as they rose above us, at my delighted love for the small boy beside me, at the sight of Rebecca trying not to glare across the aisle, having spent the flight looking after a five-year-old: what storms of neurotransmission, reception and processing were these! And all manifesting as a look of self-absorbed detachment on my face as I stared out of the window. No wonder *Translational Psychiatry* describes our knowledge of the neurobiology of dysfunction as 'rudimentary'.

This makes it less surprising when Peter Macrae explains that treatments are matched to mood disorders by trial and error.

'The only reason to choose one over another is the side effects. You can't really know. Aripiprazole is supposed to be special, with fewer side effects. Clozapine works when others haven't,' Peter says. 'You can use it for drug-resistant psychosis, but there's some reluctance to prescribing it and to taking it, because you need a blood test regularly – weekly – and you can never stop monitoring. It can lead to agranulocytosis – the bone marrow stops making white blood cells.'

The distress I feel at the thought of people facing lifetimes of daily pills and weekly blood tests must cross my face.

'But I've seen these drugs working,' Peter says. 'I've seen all of them working.'

Now he talks about the growth in alternative treatments, suggesting that the future will be much less about the prescription of drugs and much more about different forms of social prescribing (which is when your doctor suggests you should get out more, take up exercise and hobbies and immerse yourself in nature) and about therapies involving art, literature, writing, music and creativity.

'Art therapies, social prescribing, conversations based on "How are you? What are you worried about? What is not right in your world?"' Peter says. '*That's* where I begin now.'

His demeanour changes. While he was describing the dopamine and other hypotheses, he seemed sombre, apparently vexed by the combination of briefing me on the complexity of the brain and our current state of acute scientific uncertainty as to what actually happens inside it. But the prospect of art therapies, social prescribing and treatments which start with patients' individual circumstances, feelings and pressures animates and enthuses him.

'It's about trying to treat people in terms of their worries and needs, from relationships to employment and social situations,' Peter says.

I bring us back to my case, asking if there is a conventional set of delusions to which the manic and psychotic are prone. What do our delusions reveal about the ways in which we are suffering, and about the ways in which we might be treated?

'It tends to be the big themes of the time,' he says. 'Back in the day, people might have believed they were being persecuted by the king. You find very exotic, creative delusions. And you get ideas attached to certain celebrities, the Internet and social media, obviously, and shadowy elements, technology spying on you, governments, MI5, the Illuminati, alien abduction.

'Sometimes people feel they have to draw connections between different spheres – it's the protection of the sense of identity. Psychology and biology are the same thing. We know cognitive behavioural therapy has neurochemical effects. It's easy to understand the categorical thinking [of the mind in crisis]: reality is all overlaps and nuances.'

I grin ruefully, thinking of my delusions about a great undertaking that would solve all the world's problems, but this is crucial. *Psychology and biology are the same thing*: a mental breakdown is also a physical crisis. The malnutrition, drugs, sleeplessness and stress of my time of chaos would have driven anyone I know to crisis. I believe I was able to hold out partly because of the high morale imparted by my delusions. I had immense purpose, driven by the certainty of my role in a scheme of unquestionable significance. I felt secure about my place within the system I created and was thus free to act with confidence. I was liberated from the grey areas, uncertainties and subtleties of reality. No wonder I felt I could do anything. Peter's 'categorical thinking' describes my case exactly, along with the connections I made between different spheres of delusion, and the absolute way I believed and defended them.

'What do we know about what really works in the treatment of psychosis?' I ask. The answer astonishes me.

'The outcomes for psychosis are better in Third World societies than they are here,' Peter says. 'Meaningful support. There are more closely knit and supportive communities in the non-industrialised world than there are in Western societies.'

This seems extraordinary. The NHS spent £12.2 billion on mental health in 2018–19, including treatments for psychosis, more than the gross domestic products of at least seventy developing countries. But it seems our wards, our psychiatrists and our drug treatments do not help people to recover from breakdown as effectively as membership of societies in which individuals are less isolated.

'And what of the future?' I ask.

'In the next decade genomics is going to be the big thing. Your DNA profile may give us 230 genes which carry risk factors, which may contribute to five or six genes which are associated with mood disorders. That will lead to much more personalised treatments – we may be able to match medications and genes via a blood test. But that leads you to questions about sinister insurance profiling, for example. How will you control who has access to your information? In the next few decades a great deal of money is going to be made in genetic profiling and matching treatments – bespoke and expensive treatments. What you hope is that the cutting edge of these technologies will be freely available on the NHS, but . . .'

The implication is clear. The very rich may be set fair for bespoke gene-based treatments. The rest of us can only live in hope.

It is time for Peter Macrae to get back to recovering from the operation on his appendix – a vigorous business, it seems. With a handshake and a grin he launches himself into the currents of London.

I leave our encounter mulling what I have learned. There is no chemical imbalance in my brain, or if there is, we have no way of identifying it. According to this consultant psychiatrist – out of the three I have met the one who gave me the most time – my conviction that the breakdown was triggered by cannabis and stress is 'a fair shout'; it is not unlikely. I could take pills, but their prescription will be based on trial and error and side effects. Judging by the ways in which Peter Macrae now frames his treatments, the most important ways forward are good, close relationships, a supportive environment, a balanced and harmonious approach to work and strong roles for music, literature, art and creativity.

I am fortunate at work and at home. My university employers are absolutely understanding. That my department is a collection of writers and poets seems to lend an edge of deep sympathy to its approach to management. The poet and professor John McAuliffe draws up a timetable which gives me months to read, write and recover, while easing me back into supervision and marking duties. My colleagues are supremely kind. Honor Gavin and Ian McGuire covered my marking during the breakdown. They wave my thanks away. Another colleague, a tremendous writer and scholar, tells her own story of depression. 'It's really nothing to worry about,' she says. 'They covered for me, we cover for you – that's how it works.' Professor Jeanette Winterson sits me down. 'I know,' she says as I start to tell her what happened. 'I know all about it. I know about the marking, I know about the breakdown. We're here for you. You're feeling better? Good. So get better and come back.' Her memoir *Why Be Happy When You Could Be Normal?* tells the story of a terrifying breakdown and a mighty recovery, effected without doctors but by walking, eating, sleeping, writing and a profound coming-to-terms with trauma.

Of this period at home, Rebecca says, 'I don't know how it happened really, but after Kenya you just came back into the house.' I try to be very respectful of the ways in which the house has changed in my absence. Robin now has the main bedroom: he is six foot five and no other room in the house will accommodate him. Our little boy has Robin's old room. There is a standing joke in the family that I hate IKEA and regard a trip there as a grievous assault on one's mental well-being. But Rebecca is a fan, and so we go and come back with a bed for our boy which Rebecca puts together. She cannot bear anyone else to interfere when she has a flat-pack to play with. She has converted the attic, formerly my writing room, into her bedroom. Very gradually, it comes to be known as our bedroom. For a long, long time I do not ask for a key to the front door.

Our son, now six, seems entirely at home in his life and with his parents. Rebecca and I argue sometimes, and at other times we hug, and when our boy finds us doing this in the kitchen he puts his arms around our legs and we all hug. He raises the crisis only once. We are in the car (I have replaced the crashed Toyota).

'Dad?'

'Yes, darling?'

'You know when you crashed the other car into the reservoir?'

'Yes . . . well, I didn't actually crash it into the reservoir. I was driving and I got ill and the car rolled down a bank and crashed at the bottom. I wasn't inside it; I jumped out.'

'So you didn't crash the car into the reservoir?'

'No. I didn't.'

'Well,' he says after a thoughtful pause, 'I've been telling people you did.' The line is delivered in a satisfied, resolved tone. I do not know what has been said to him about the period of my absence. He was accustomed to me going away for work. The only time I ask Rebecca about it, about what she told him when we were separated and fighting, and I was mad, she says, 'I told him about the bad wolf and the good wolf.'

'What do you mean?'

'I said, well, you have a bad wolf and a good wolf inside you, and if you feed the good wolf things go well, and you are happy, and you make people happy – and if you feed the bad wolf you get into trouble and hurt people and they don't want to be with you. I told him you had been feeding the bad wolf. He understood completely. He's cool about it.'

I think of the drugs, the grandiose plans, the refusal to address the illness, the ranging around, the egotism, the lies. Feeding the bad wolf: yes, I did do that. And I am feeding the good wolf now, almost exclusively, except for my lies about the pills.

Living the lies is awful. Having been a cannabis addict and a cheat, I am familiar with the mental calculations of the liar. When asked or challenged I keep my cool and as easily as I can I say the words: 'Yes, I've taken my pill.'

Somewhere in my soul it feels as though I am shelling out a payment from an empty account, defrauding something deep inside me. With each lie I am renewing a promise that there is a reason for this – that the future will redeem this present somehow; that there is a higher purpose. I tell myself the violence against myself is worse than the deception I am practising on Rebecca or my mother or whoever asks me about the pills – and I can feel it. The feeling is like the tightening of a sore little screw. Only days or months or years later, when I am found out or when I confess, will I realise what it really was that I spent each time. It was freedom. Each lie takes a little freedom with it, a little more space and peace, a little ease.

The guilt, the lie, I shift into a shadow version of me, my mangy twin. I tell myself I am not a bad person, a liar, a cheat, not really; I am simply in the position of having to wear a mask. I give all the guilt to this dented version of myself and I keep him well out of sight – as far out of my own sight as possible. My shadow is stitched together like a rag doll of patches of guilt, humiliation and shame. Meanwhile, I am the front man. I regret it and I carry on. It will not be this way for ever, I tell myself, but it has to be this way now.

Compared to other lies I have told – no, I'm not smoking dope; no I'm not sleeping with anyone else – this one was easy. I wish I had not done it. I wish I had not felt I had to do it. But so it was.

There are moments of shivering uncertainty. I find myself standing in the living room of the flat one day, holding a sheet of unopened aripiprazole pills and talking to myself.

'Are you quite sane?'

I do not feel quite sane. I feel shaky and entirely alone. There is no one to talk to: for the first time in my life I feel there is not one friend I can confide in, who would understand. Given that I was in a mental hospital a few months ago, which of them is not going to tell me to take the pills?

'If you're not sane, you should take one,' I advise myself.

But I am not high, and not depressed. I am tremulous, uncertain, bereft of confidence and lonely. *See how it goes*, I decide. Get through the day, eat and sleep, keep a steady course, keep up the front, the happy and capable front. Things will get better. And if they don't, go back on the pills.

Things do get better. Having this book to research and plan helps enormously. Rebecca's rhythm, the long walks on the moors, the meals in the Packhorse – our favourite pub, up on Widdop Moor, near where I crashed the car – bring us together and lift me out of myself. She and our boy and I, and the dog, cover miles at the weekends. We drift along, chatting, stopping to talk to horses, greet swallows and observe rabbits. I have never really understood the concept of mindfulness but the practice of being in the moment, being engaged with what is before you and around you, releasing the gnawing tugs of the past and the stalking cares of the future in exchange for a feeling of the fullness of the present, I do understand, at least when we are outside. Perhaps mindfulness just means mooching along, looking at what is, as your thoughts come and go gently. All my life I have watched birds and stared at views. Did I not realise how rich and necessary that was – did I forget?

One Sunday afternoon we make a great loop, up through the woods to the moor, along the ridges to Widdop, pausing at the Packhorse, which is shut, and return via the long lane to Heptonstall. Our valley lies below us, the fields running down to treetops where the ground plunges steeply towards the stream. It is a temperate summer day, that lovely timeless period between afternoon and evening. The stone walls, the sky, the meadows and the dozing farms have an eternal aspect. We could be walking through the years of my childhood, or my parents' time. Perhaps it is only this that I crave, I think, watching the little boy as he feeds a horse over a fence, and Rebecca watches him with such love, and a notation of swallows on a telegraph wire watch us all. Yes. This is happiness. This is fortune. This is wealth.

CHAPTER 29

How we got here

Being diagnosed as bipolar and spending time in a psychiatric institution had a powerful effect on my idea of myself and my understanding of where I stood in society. It is like being given a new citizenship: suddenly you are part of a new country, with its own history, laws, customs and expectations. You belong to a secret sect which exists everywhere, hiding in the open. Sometimes I thought of my experiences as akin to a travel writing job which went horribly wrong. When friends asked about it, I told them that it was as though I had been to a strange, remote place where disasters had befallen me; it was like coming back from a journey which I had been lucky to survive. It was a comforting story to tell them and myself but it was too pat, too convenient an explanation: journeys end, but nothing I read or felt suggested that I would be able to leave the madness and its consequences behind.

Unexpected, unwanted citizenship is a better metaphor. As I strengthened, as my sense of hope and agency became less tremulous, I began to explore this new country, seeking to discover how it came about, and what my place in it might be.

Michel Foucault saw madness as 'a phenomenon of civilisation, as variable, as floating as any other phenomenon of culture'; curing the mad, he concluded, 'is not the only possible reaction to the phenomenon of madness'. Foucault, among others, regarded the rise of the modern objectifying approach to madness as a means of social control, the othering of a threat to the rise of the mercantile bourgeois family. In the Middle Ages madness was treated like leprosy: you were sick or healthy, you enjoyed reason or suffered unreason. With the Renaissance came more nuanced thinking. As Shakespeare's Theseus observes, 'The lunatic, the lover and the poet / Are of imagination all compact': degrees of passion and disturbance flow through many lives at many times. Madness was explored as a form of knowledge, an insight akin to religious experience. But societies of the seventeenth and eighteenth centuries saw reason and madness as strictly separable opposites. Institutions were built, and the insane – those who, as professionals would now say, 'presented' anomalously – were confined. Romantic and humanist thinkers questioned this separation. Madness began to be seen less as a tragic state than a critical position: the world is more mad than the lunatic, who is simply pointing this out. The mad belong to the edges of the world's reason, and they expose the limits of reason's world, suggest the works of Montaigne, Rabelais, Gogol and Erasmus. These writers delighted in demarcating and exposing the difference between what people are and what they pretend to be. Their characters expose the everyday 'madness' of the world we accept as a natural part of reality (institutionalised venality, injustice, corruption, leadership by thugs, brutes and maniacs, etc).

The lights that the mad have thrown upon their societies, and the ways in which societies have treated them, are fascinating. The psychiatrist Joanna Moncrieff has studied the history of the asylum in Britain. She cites the work of sociologist and historian of psychiatry Andrew Scull. Scull, Moncrieff writes, 'suggests that the asylums were part of a broader system of social welfare and control, under the umbrella of the Poor Law in England, and linked with the workhouse (and its equivalent elsewhere). The workhouse was designed to force the "able-bodied" poor into work, and the asylums developed as a specialist alternative for people who were unfit for this plan.'

Moncrieff's study of hundreds of case histories leads her to surprising conclusions: 'Modern treatments can effectively suppress some symptoms, which may reduce the time people need to spend in an institution, but it is not clear that current recovery rates are any better than they were at the beginning of the 20th century.'

I remember first hearing the phrase, 'Care in the Community' in the 1980s. A man on my father's street in north London was shouting and raving. 'That's Care in the Community,' Dad said. It meant deinstitutionalisation, brought about partly by exposure of the poor management of asylums and inadequate treatment of their inhabitants, partly by a political desire to cap spending on long-stay care, and partly by a conviction that care of the mentally ill in their own homes, funded by local authorities, rather than in asylums, would serve them better. In the public mind the asylum, mental hospital or 'loony bin' was a strange and fearful place. Children, certainly those with whom I was at school in Wales and Worcestershire, knew the names of their local hospitals and used them as taunts and teases. But Joanna Moncrieff finds that, from the sufferers' perspective, these institutions did not deserve their reputation.

Asylums were clearly places where people who were unable to look after themselves or were disturbing the peace, for reasons of organic disease or psychological disturbance, were sequestered until such time as they recovered their health or their sanity. The asylum system was founded on the belief

that it could restore people to sanity, and regular inspections
were designed to maintain these goals and ensure the quality
of care.

Discoveries were made in the more enlightened asylums but
came to be neglected in favour of the heavy medication of
mental illness. In *The Well-Gardened Mind*, the psychiatrist
and gardener Sue Stuart-Smith writes: 'In 1812 Benjamin
Rush, an American physician who was one of the founding
fathers of the United States, published a manual on the
treatment of mental illness. In it, he observed that mental
health patients who worked in the asylum grounds because
they needed to pay for their care by cutting wood, making
fires, and digging in the garden often made the best recov-
eries. In contrast, those of higher social status were more
likely to "languish away their lives within the walls of the
hospital".'

It has taken twenty years of the twenty-first century for
this insight to return with strength. Progressive doctors, such
as the GP who treated the journalist Isabel Hardman, now
ask questions about their patients' outdoor activities and their
access to green spaces, urging sufferers to walk, run, swim
– whatever it takes to get us out of our rooms. Doctors now
see a role for nature in what until recently has been an almost
entirely medicated space. Hardman was suffering from
PTSD, depression, anxiety, paranoia and suicidal ideation.
Although she was treated with antidepressants, her GP also
'listened, and told me that I should arrange riding lessons
and running sessions that it would be hard to duck out of',
she writes in her book *The Natural Health Service*.

It seems certain that we will see more and more of just
the sort of social prescribing favoured by Peter Macrae, as
it comes to be widely understood that it is both effective and
cost-effective. However, the story of the treatment of
madness, from the time of Benjamin Rush to our own, twists

and turns away from nature and other therapies, towards
medication.

The condition from which I have been told I suffer, bipolar
disorder, did not exist in the early twentieth century. A
hundred years ago I might have been diagnosed with manic
depression or told I had suffered a nervous breakdown. My
prospects would have been good: a study in 1929 of 2000
manic depressive patients, run by Johns Hopkins medical
school in the United States, found that 80 per cent recovered
within a year and fewer than 1 per cent needed prolonged
treatment in hospital.

In 1931, 50 per cent of people who were treated for mania
in the mental hospitals of New York State suffered no second
episode. The case for manic depression as a rare illness with
good chances for recovery would seem to have been proved
by Ming Tsuang of the University of Iowa, who followed
the fortunes of 86 people hospitalised for manic breakdown
between 1935 and 1944. Tsuang studied this group over 30
years. Some 70 per cent had good outcomes: they fully reinte-
grated into society, work and familial relationships. Over the
period Tsuang studied, half showed no symptoms at all.

These studies are cited by Robert Whitaker in his book
*Anatomy of an Epidemic: Magic Bullets, Psychiatric Drugs, and
the Astonishing Rise of Mental Illness in America*. Whitaker is
a renowned figure in a movement which opposes the widespread use of psychiatric drugs, holding that a sinister and
damaging alliance between pharmaceutical corporations and
psychiatrists is responsible for the mass medication of the
unwell. The movement maintains that the chemical treatment
of mental illness is vastly profitable to Big Pharma and to
psychiatry, and is a model which produces short-term benefit
at the cost of huge long-term harm. Whether or not you
agree with him, Whitaker is a scrupulous journalist and
researcher: his sources are verifiable and his reports, if not
his conclusions, are unquestioned.

One might ask if the average manic depressive of the 1920s and 30s can be usefully compared to a bipolar-diagnosed individual now. I am certain my generation has taken more illegal drugs, for example, than did our grandparents' generation, and recovery rates of 70 and 80 per cent make an arresting contrast to our own time. The *Harvard Mental Health Letter*, published by Harvard Medical School, stated in 2008: 'in a study of people with bipolar disorder type 1, characterised by episodes of mania (rather than hypomania) with or without depression, researchers followed [medicated] patients after they suffered a manic or depressive episode. They found that 37 per cent of patients experienced a recurrence of mania or depression within a year, 60 per cent within two years, and 73 per cent within five years.'

Something would seem to have changed for the worse. The anti-psychiatry movement blames the rise of psychiatric drugs, along with the chemical-imbalance theory of mental illness. The question of psychiatric drugs remains vexed, but since my conversation with Peter Macrae I have learned more about the chemical-imbalance theory. In *Great Myths of the Brain* Christian Jarret describes its inception. In 1967 researchers Joseph Schildkraut and Seymour Kety proposed a link between emotional states and levels of monoamine neurotransmitters (norepinephrine and, later, serotonin). 'These pioneers were careful not to attribute an exclusive causal role to brain chemistry,' Jarrett writes, and quotes Schildkraut and Kety: 'Any comprehensive formulation of the physiology of affective state will have to include many other concomitant biochemical, physiological and psychological factors.'

'Despite their caution,' Jarrett writes, 'the chemical imbalance myth took hold.'

Did it ever. Let us leave aside for a moment questions of corporate profit-hunger, marketing budgets and psychiatry's desire to stand on an equal footing with other branches of medicine, all of which are loudly proclaimed by the anti-psychiatry movement. The scenario in the treatment rooms of the 1950s and 60s was fundamentally identical to what I experienced in my encounters with Dr X and Dr Y. In both situations, you have a patient who is – or was very recently – seriously unwell, and a doctor with the power to prescribe pills or injections which have a verifiable beneficial effect, at least in the short term. (We will return to the question of long-term consequences.) Crucially, just like Dr X and Dr Y, like thousands of psychiatrists, the doctors of the 1950s and 60s lacked alternative treatments. What would you do in their shoes? Unless you were radically opposed to conventional psychiatric drugs (and some, like R. D. Laing, who had more faith in LSD than antipsychotics, were) and prepared to face the consequences of non-prescription, which might include breakdown or suicide, leading to the coroner's court, where you would be asked to explain your decisions, you would prescribe, of course.

The era of psychiatric medication began in the 1950s. Chlorpromazine, branded Thorazine in the United States and Largactil in Europe, was approved for prescription in the US in 1954. 'Thirteen months later it was being given to two million people in that country alone,' writes Andrew Scull in *Madness and Civilisation*. Scull describes the new landscape of mental health treatment: 'Most psychiatrists hailed the therapeutic breakthrough they claimed this represented. Instead of relying on crude empirical treatments including the various shock therapies, or the even cruder surgical intervention that was lobotomy, the profession could now prescribe and administer that classic symbolic accoutrement of the modern physician – drugs.'

Where the anti-psychiatry movement now sees conspiracy, what happened next can also be framed as a simple story of market forces. We know that mental disorders can spring from any number of causes: childhood trauma, unhappy relationships, unemployment or trouble at work, drug use, bereavement, abuse, painful life events, head or other injury, exposure to poverty, war or any of the anxieties which might beset an ordinary life. The number and range of these afflictions produce a huge demand for treatment. Drug companies provide the supply. The psychiatrist puts the two together. What does it matter if there is no chemical imbalance in the brain? Drug companies promote the narrative anyway: it is easy to grasp (if not to understand) and it offers a solution. The psychiatrist prescribes, and the patient, gratefully, takes the pills, in hope and expectation. If they were not effective we would surely not be in our current position: over 70 million prescriptions for anti-depressants in the UK every year, and climbing, with 7.3 million people taking them in 2018, 4.4 million of whom had taken them for at least two years. In 2016, one in six Americans took a psychiatric drug: antidepressants were the most common, followed by anti-anxiety medication, with antipsychotics in third place.

The question, though, is what we mean by 'effective'.

Here the story becomes vexed. Even among those professionals who are most suspicious of psychiatric drugs, there is a general recognition that they can and do help in the short term. No one denies that they alleviate symptoms. When those symptoms include delusions, paranoia and manic behaviour, it takes a very brave (or foolish) clinician to argue against the prescription of psychiatric drugs, although such people do exist, in growing numbers, as we shall see.

The disputed area is what happens next, in the medium to long term. In 2018 the *New York Times* reported: 'While the drugs have helped millions of people with depression and anxiety, and many people can stop taking them without significant issues, some individuals who try to wean themselves off cannot due to harsh withdrawal symptoms they say they were not warned of. Initially, the drugs were cleared for short-term use; but even today, with millions of long-term users, there is little data about their effects on individuals who take them for years.'

There may be no underlying chemical imbalance for the drugs to 'fix', but the act of taking them surely creates one – hence the withdrawal symptoms. Writing for the *Psychiatric Times* in 2011, Donald Goff reviewed three long-term studies of the effects of antipsychotics on the brain, two on humans and one on monkeys. Goff concludes: 'Taken together, these studies suggest that antipsychotics may contribute to early gray matter loss and, later in the course of treatment, to white matter loss. These effects may be dose-related and probably are not prevented by the use of second-generation agents. This argues for minimising antipsychotic exposure both acutely and long-term.' Goff goes on to note that psychosis, left to itself, also seems to cause brain damage. 'Longer DUP [duration of untreated psychosis] has been associated with poorer symptomatic and functional outcomes as well as brain volume loss.'

Despite rejecting clinical advice to take lithium or aripiprazole, then, and not now suffering any symptoms of mania or depression, I am in a good place by the early summer. (I am, however, feeling rather nervous about upcoming engagements at literary festivals, and am shaky in myself, deep down.) I am not taking psychiatric drugs, so not suffering side effects or facing the prospect of withdrawal symptoms. Those pills I have taken seem to have helped do the job that the ward and the mental health services exist to do: I am back on my feet, out in the world and functioning.

The one fixed point in my calendar, every year since 2003, has been the Hay Festival, which falls in the last week of May and the first week of June. I am due to perform at several events and I am chairing several more. Hay can be a slightly terrifying prospect, because I love it so much that I get nervous about not giving it my best shot. But it is always an enchanted highlight of the year, a vivid, inspiring time in a special place, where I am guaranteed to meet many of the people I most like and most admire in the world. The festival's organisers, the crews and their audiences have seen my whole life as a writer. Professionally, I was born and grew up on these stages, in these tents. Every time I take the road to Hay it feels like both a homecoming and an advance into new territory. I have friends here, people I feel I know well, oddly, as we only meet once a year. The heightened feeling of festival time seems to make all its moments more intense.

There is Jenny, who runs the catering in the Green Room, with her wise kind smile. There is George, who works in the backstage crew, who is about as wild as I was at his age. There is Maisie who looks after the artists, whom I always ask for gossip, which is rarely given: she works for *Private Eye*. At the BBC tents are old friends and colleagues among the producers and engineers. It all gives me the strangest, strongest sense of belonging. Convening us all, and miraculously, though unimaginably busy, never seeming rushed, are Becky Shaw and Peter Florence. We hug. Peter has me down for a dozen events this year. I take it as a vote of complete faith: you say you are ready to work? Here you are, then. Show them . . .

When the family of writers meets, often in green rooms and the backstage spaces of festivals, there is a reliable subtext in the question 'How's it going?' It means 'How are you in yourself? How is the book going? What are you writing next? How are the family? How is your mental health?' Madness, depression, anxiety and mania are not uncommon in the profession, and have been discussed openly among us for decades.

I meet Frank Cottrell-Boyce in the Green Room. He is a hero of mine, dressed today in a white suit.

'How's it going, Frank?'

'Well,' he says quietly, with a grin, 'we're not digging coal, are we?'

I am chairing Robert Macfarlane, who is in the middle of launching his new book, *Underland*. He is the most modest star moving easily in an environment which all of us know, which we need and love on some level (and dread on another) but which you never quite get used to: being on show, with eyes on you, swinging between the adrenaline of the performance and the comedown of the aftermath.

'How's it going, Rob?'

'I shouldn't complain, it sounds terrible, but I got sent the timetable for my US tour and it's horrific – completely relentless! I'm absolutely dreading it. I keep thinking, just get through it . . . just *get through it* and then you can go home . . . But how are you? How's Rebecca? How's the book?'

He knows about the breakdown. Back at the end of March we walked together in Scotland over a long weekend. He coaxed me up half a dozen Munros. On the last day, as we descended a series of icy ridges, I explained what had happened. A friend of his had something similar and worse happen to him, so Rob has seen psychosis close up. I tell him about the book. He pauses. 'In mountaineering,' he says, 'when you get lost, you can follow your footprints through snow. Even if it's a while afterwards and the snow has melted, you can follow your tracks because the compacted snow melts at a different rate – your prints actually stand up, they're raised. Perhaps what you are doing is like that – following your raised prints back to find yourself.'

Yes, I think, *exactly* – as Zaffar Kunial put it, hunting the ghost of yourself.

In the garden behind the Green Room is Kapka Kassabova, here to talk about her book *Border*.

'I've written a very strange book about a lake,' she says. 'I don't know if anyone will read it. But it was a kind of healing. How are you?'

I explain. We have known each other for a long time, though only met properly once, when we taught for a week together at a writing centre in Scotland. Kapka gives the impression of never having said anything stupid or unconsidered. She reminds me of my Russian teacher at school, who was, like Kapka, also Bulgarian. A deeply serious intelligence regards you from a gaze in which joy and a kind of melancholy are intermingled. She is tremendously easy to talk to – part of the secret of her books is the way people talk to her, astonishingly openly and intimately, on short acquaintance. I pour out my story.

Kapka understands. She was physically ill, she says; what I imagined must have been a wonderful year touring *Border* was, in her body and mind, a cruel and frightening time. Writing *To the Lake* (which turns out to be a triumph) was part of a necessary healing, as she describes it, a gruelling pursuit of stories and meanings alongside a prolonged and urgent search for health in her body and balance in her soul. We talk about soul, spirit and the physical. 'I got there,' she said. 'I am worried no one will read the book but I am in a good place. I found a good teacher, a great man. You will get there. But it takes work. It takes a lot of *self-work*, and you have to accept that, and you have to do it.'

These three conversations – we're not digging coal, follow your footprints back to find yourself, and do the self-work – I take with me from Hay. They become part of my mantra in the following months. And one other thing: in the Green Room the rapper and poet Rufus Mufasa is incredibly kind, bursting with encouragement and support. One of the reasons Peter Florence, the festival's father, loves Hay is the Green Room, the cross-currents of connection and conversation between writers from different worlds all suddenly presented with our own odd kind. Many people feel like freaks some of the time. Writers are particularly prone to it. Hay assures you, gleefully, that you not alone, that your odd and quixotic and difficult existence is a rich and honourable profession, and that your peers are like you and with you and everywhere, however little you see of them. Rufus gives me a beautiful notebook. 'Here you are!' she says. 'Do something wonderful with it.'

CHAPTER 30

The front line

The self-work Kapka advocated I set about in two ways: with my therapist, with whom suddenly I begin to make progress, and in the fashion Rob advocated, following my footprints back through what happened. So I talk to the people who dealt with me, in order better to understand the system which treats many thousands like me.

I make an assumption in every encounter with these people, one I have held since first coming across what seemed and seems a widespread and growing crisis in mental health: that more of us are suffering more unhappiness, trauma and distress, from anxiety to breakdown, more of the time. But is there actually a crisis in mental health, and if so, what is its shape?

That the world's mental health is in severe difficulty seems unarguable. A 2018 study by the Lancet Commission identified a 'global crisis' which is causing 'a monumental loss of human capabilities, and avoidable suffering'. 'The global burden of disease attributable to mental disorders has risen in all countries in the context of major demographic, environmental, and socio-political transitions,' the commission reported. Homing in on the underfunding of services for children and adolescents, 'arguably the most important developmental phase in the context of prevention', the report said, 'The economic consequences of this low investment are staggering, with an estimated loss of US$16 trillion to the global economy due to mental disorders (in the period 2010–30), driven in part by the early age of onset and loss of productivity across the life course.'

The Institute of Health Metrics Evaluation calculates that around 971 million people, 13 per cent of the global population, are suffering from some sort of mental disorder, with dementia the fastest rising. However, the IHME denies that the richest countries are experiencing a critical expansion in rates of mental illness, which it says are growing no faster than their populations. The growth, it seems, is in the popular experience of mental illness, due perhaps to destigmatisation, certainly to a greater willingness to report and seek help for problems, and unquestionably to the number of people taking medication. The use of antidepressants has doubled in Britain in the last ten years, as it has throughout the developed world. At the same time, UK rates of detention under the Mental Health Act have increased by 34 per cent in a decade. Campaigners suspect this may be because patients are released too quickly, in order to free up beds, leading to repeated detentions. The number of those suffering the severest forms of mental illness has also climbed.

So while our experience of mental illness is much expanded – we hear, see and think more about it, we know people who suffer from it and people who take pills related to it – there is not a rocketing rate of suffering (assuming the IHME is correct). But there are two unfolding crises in mental health treatment in Britain today. The first is in the allocation of resources. While 23 per cent of the activity of the National Health Service is taken up by dealing with mental illness, only 11 per cent of its funding goes to mental health trusts.

The second is the disaster befalling our children and adolescents. Teachers and doctors report that anxiety, depression, self-harm, eating disorders and addiction are rife and rising among the young. In the last two years, according to teachers surveyed by the National Education Union, the well-being of pupils has deteriorated. Eighty-three per cent of those surveyed had witnessed an increase in numbers of children needing help. Their schools had little or no means of giving it, they said. Seventy per cent of teachers said they had no school nurse, and the same percentage had found no means of accessing NHS support for their pupils. Fewer than half said their school had a counsellor. The Association of Child Psychotherapists calls the situation 'a silent catastrophe', the title of the organisation's 2018 report into mental health provision for young people. The problem, it says, is the destruction of NHS child and adolescent mental health provision. The disappearance of specialist services, fragmentation and underfunding caused by competitive tendering, redesigned services which no longer meet their users' needs, chronic shortages of time and money for assessment and treatment, shattered staff morale, the closure of senior posts, raised thresholds for treatment – the report makes sickening reading. The Children's Commissioner for England, Anne Longfield, estimates it will cost £10 billion to fix what she calls 'the broken safety net' for vulnerable children. Meanwhile, the Department for Health and Social Care and the Department for Education both claimed, in 2019, that an extra £2.3 billion a year will go to mental health support for children.

When I talked to the police, to health executives, to leaders of local government, to nurses and social workers, I asked each about 'the crisis in mental health'. None demurred at the term: a rising demand for services, particularly among the young, the old and the poor; forecasts of a doubling in the cost of mental health provision in the next twenty years; present and projected cuts; a system scrambling to adjust and struggling to cope (and all this before the effects of Covid-19 are factored in) is surely a crisis. The disaster caused by the virus is leading to a further increased need for mental health services. Across the entire spectrum, more people are in difficulty: rates of everything from anxiety to psychosis have jumped and are climbing. Combine this with recession, the contraction of the labour market (it was established during the financial crisis of 2008 that job losses and suicide rates rise together) and the economic price of Brexit, and it seems certain that we will, as a society, break new ground in the widespread experience of mental suffering in the next few years.

At the same time, though, the Covid-19 crisis has shown what can be done to help, and has speeded the doing of it. The NHS was already planning to offer many more mental health services remotely, by phone, app and through online meetings. Provisions which were scheduled to take a year or more to implement were in some areas rolled out in weeks in 2020, in response to the leap in demand. A raised awareness of the need to take care of our minds, crumbling taboos around admitting to the experience of mental illness, and new ways of thinking about it and treating it combine to suggest there are shafts of light and hope in the otherwise hard and sombre times to come. Whatever happens, the men and women who are the faces of the agencies and institutions which dealt with me will be the first to feel it.

When someone breaks down, GPs, NHS staff in accident and emergency departments and the police are usually the first to deal with them.

With me it was the police, so I go to Halifax to meet Chief Superintendent Dickie Whitehead, whose responsibility I was, unwittingly, each time his officers had dealings with me. The chief superintendent is a trim, spry man, his white hair clipped short, his shoes as shiny as a general's. He wears his close-fitting uniform like combat gear: it emerges that he was in the Royal Navy before he joined the police. Pale blue eyes take you in in a flicker and fix you with a look somewhere between toughness and compassion. The voice is large, as Yorkshire as Halifax stone, and the manners are immaculate.

I ask him about his work in the Calder Valley.

'What is the policing mission?' he returns. As he speaks, I realise with delight that Dickie Whitehead is a natural teacher, in love with his job. 'It's the protection of life and limb, and my focus is the front line. That's my true north. When I speak to my officers here in Halifax I keep it very simple. Is what we do fit for family – for your family? Is the service we are providing, is the way I am behaving fit for my family? Because if it is fit for my family then it is fit for our community.'

'What happens when they find themselves dealing with mental health cases?'

'Often we pick people up – people in the situation you were in, perhaps – and we have to use a police station as a place of safety. But it's the last and worst place you should ever be. In the last two or three years we have started to wake up to a new understanding. We now have a mental health nurse working alongside the officers in the station on lates and nights. The nurse makes assessments about what the issues are. And then, depending on the situation, if someone's unwell the ambulance service can come and convey them to somewhere they can be treated. But if there are risks then we will provide an escort. And I don't have the resilience in my budget to have two officers tied up escorting someone to hospital for four or five hours. It can happen that the hospital doesn't have the ability to receive them. Then you've got front-line police officers sitting in a van.'

I asked the Chief Superintendent how things have changed for the police as the crisis in mental health has grown.

'There's been a sea-change in emphasis based on safe-guarding against threat, harm and risk. There are the elderly, there are vulnerable adults, we get children absconding from care – and at the same time we've had a comprehensive spending review which reduced officer numbers. Not as much is being in invested in policing.'

'Do your officers have training in dealing with people who are mad rather than bad?' I ask.

'Training?' he booms. 'No, I wouldn't say we had training. We have inputs. We have guidance for attending the Dales Ward.'

The Dales is a local mental hospital.

'What are the inputs?'

'Well, we talk about it among ourselves. We debrief. We discuss what's happened.'

Chief Superintendent Whitehead's face takes on a cast which is both mischievous and enthusiastic.

'Look, my officers are trained in the escalation of use of force. If there's a risk of violence then my cops can use the baton on yer, gas yer, get the cuffs on and get yer in the van. If there's an escalation of violence then that's what's going to happen. We're trained in communication skills. We try to talk someone round and talk them down before you have to lay hands on. But how to support someone in crisis is not widely known. It takes a real understanding and awareness of language. And it depends on time and place. When you've got someone on the bridge, we have trained negotiators and influencers, but by the time we get that person there, often they've either gone off themselves or we've got them down. Then our first priority is to get an assessment. Ideally we'd get annual mental health training for dealing with the acute mental health crisis. Look at the NYPD. They looked at their management of calls and they realised a lot of the complaints were around landlords, disputes between neighbours, so they directed all those calls to the housing associations. That could work – one clearing house for calls for public-sector services.'

As he talks I am seeing again the insides of police cars and vans; the mill of officers behind the desk in the station in the small hours, the calm, matter-of-fact way they treated me, the kindness behind the *clink* and *click* of their cuffs and batons. The tough, eager, front-foot approach of their boss makes perfect sense of the way they behaved towards me, the immaculate way they treated Rebecca and all of us who were involved in this story. They are indeed fit for family.

'What about the strain on your officers? Presumably the police are also seeing an increase in mental health issues?'

'We're the one emergency service no one want to see,' he says with mordant satisfaction. 'We have got an increase in stress and we do pay more attention to safeguarding and counselling. In fact my force has some of the best and lowest sickness levels in the country. A lot of work is done through the inspectors and through the sergeants. The message is, it's good to talk, to suggest that someone might want to go and talk to Occupational Health. A sergeant might suggest an officer goes to a doctor to talk about mental health.'

'What are your worries, personally?'

'There's an increase in the number of officers off with stress. There's a definite rise in people needing our help. It can get to the point of breaking. Obviously there needs to be investment in mental health to help fix a broken system that's underfunded,' he says.

Talking to Chief Superintendent Whitehead gives a vivid picture of a man and a force robustly and sensitively engaged with the mental health needs and struggles of the community they serve. I realise my experience is only one case study, and perhaps a skewed one. As Rebecca noted throughout our ordeal, my accent, manners, class, confidence and connections mean authority tends to deal with me carefully, affording me privileges and considerations which should be universal, but are not.

The fact that the poor, those living in poor and deprived areas and the most vulnerable – children and the elderly – are disproportionately affected by disorders of the mind and spirit hotly shames our system, but it is coldly revealing. We know that having more money means better access to services. For the less well-off – those who have less experience of finding, asking for and getting what they need from society – the statistics show a huge under-exploitation of specialist services. As a result, the poorest are much more likely to end up in A & E – 70 per cent more likely in the case of poorer compared to richer teenagers. This is not just because poverty breeds illness, but because the wealthier and the better educated are 'better at making themselves heard', according to a 2007 report by the Civitas think tank. So, although the poor, the least educated and ethnic minorities visit GPs more often than the affluent and well educated, they are less likely to be referred to a specialist.

'Do not be poor, black, old and depressed in England right now, because you're very unlikely to get treated,' the report warns. There are upwards of 60,000 new detentions under the Mental Health Act every year, an increase of nearly 50 per cent over a decade ago. A government-commissioned review published in 2018 concluded, 'People with the most severe forms of mental illness have the greatest needs and continue to be the most neglected and discriminated against.' Professor Sir Simon Wessely, former head of the British College of Psychiatrists, who chaired the review, also noted, 'Experiences of people from black African and Caribbean heritage are particularly poor and they are detained more than any other group. Too often this can result in police becoming involved at time of crisis.'

The review found that many patients suffer neglect and discrimination. Many are treated without dignity or respect by staff. Professor Wessely expressed concern that the steeply climbing numbers of detentions under the Mental Health Act suggest that too many of these are taking place. The reasons for the disproportionate number of poor people and black people being sectioned are multiple but not hard to understand. For those with inadequate or no disposable incomes and deprived of equal opportunities for advancement, the stresses on mind and body are hugely increased. Access to natural environments and leisure may be greatly reduced. While the future of treatment is certain to include a much stronger focus on nature, exercise and therapies like gardening, swimming, running and walking, all these are easier to undertake for the affluent. As Isabel Hardman writes perceptively in *The Natural Health Service*, 'If you have a friend who is struggling with their mental health but really has no money at all to buy the basic items they need to go for a forest walk, then the best present you could ever give them is a pair of cheap trainers.'

When the police had done what they could with me – essentially containment and transportation to my first, fruitless, encounter with the hospital – the next service I dealt with came in the form of Lauren (not her real name), the social worker who sectioned me. I contact Lauren explaining that I am trying to understand how psychosis is diagnosed and treated, and asking if we might meet.

On a rainy summer afternoon in Halifax, warm and drippy, the sun appearing occasionally in a spill of light behind the cloud, we meet in an office in a council building in the middle of town. Lauren has brought her manager with her, a tough and kindly woman. Lauren shakes my hand. Her gaze is both kind and searching, with a still, assessing look I remember.

When she and her manager are satisfied that they understand what I am up to and assured that they will not be identified in anything I write, I ask Lauren to describe what she was doing just before we met that first time. She speaks with firmness and certainty. You can tell she is used to accounting for her actions. There is not a trace of self-doubt in her soft voice.

'I'd been doing long shifts through the night in the days before, and I'd just changed over to a day shift. I had a telephone call from the Home-Based Treatment Team and calls from the ambulance service and the police explaining what was happening and asking for advice. Your partner was expressing concern.

'What did they tell you?'

'They said you were behaving in ways that were not normal for you. The Home-Based Treatment Team didn't think that what they could do was enough. They'd had calls from the police, your brother and your partner. I remember it took quite a while to try to identify your nearest relative.

'Once I'd identified that it was your partner I had a chat and we agreed that a Mental Health Act Assessment was appropriate. I arranged for two doctors to attend. It's always an approved mental health professional who coordinates and makes the final decision, but there needs to be two doctors present, one of whom has experience with mental health treatment: a psychiatrist.

'There is no presupposition of psychosis. Street drugs or a urinary-tract infection can give a very similar presentation. So we try to rule things out. The issue for me is, the power to detain is huge. It's very intrusive, so first you try to rule out everything else.

'I contacted a couple of doctors, one of whom is always on call, and spoke to them. They were of the view it didn't sound safe to leave you on your own. Generally there is a doctor, consultant or registrar who is also a qualified psychiatrist on call. We have a lot of Section 12 doctors – that's the part of the Mental Health Act – and we all generally know each other. We do a deep-level assessment together. Someone generally leads. We all try to keep it as low key as possible. At the end we all come to our own view. We don't always agree. If both doctors are of the view a person needs help then we consider what kind of treatment would be appropriate.

I then make a final assessment. In Calderdale it's social
workers who do that. We don't just follow an assessment,
diagnosis, treatment model – a medical model. I am thinking
what is going on for this person? What alternatives to hospital
are there?'

'What sort of things do you consider?' I ask.

Lauren pauses. 'I'm thinking, what is the least restrictive
option? What are the family telling me? If the family are
saying they can't cope, is there an option that doesn't involve
detention? Is there anyone else I can talk to? Are they being
themselves? Are they just behaving in an eccentric manner?
I quite like eccentric behaviour! If they have strange beliefs,
does that mean they're well or unwell? After we talked to you
we went out to the car and had a discussion. We were all of
same view.'

'What was my case like? What did you discuss?'

'Well, you weren't very well known to mental health
services in the the area. We gathered things had been difficult
in Italy. So you have to go on what you see there and then.
How a person presents, what other people say – if you can't
evidence any risk then you wouldn't detain someone.'

'I remember the assessment very well. But what did I seem
like to you?'

'You were very genial, erudite, in many ways very
engaging. But you were avoidant of a lot of the questions;
you weren't showing an understanding of risks to yourself
and others. You were very dismissive of concerns about your
behaviour. You were dismissive of concerns about what you
were doing to your ceiling and the wires. We didn't think
you were able to weigh up the risks or options. You didn't
have the capacity to consider your care needs and risks.'

'Yes, I remember . . .'

I remember trying so hard to be normal, insisting I was
normal, rejecting hospitals and pills, trying to make my points

soberly, and yes, my hands moving, trying to explain, to fend off, to stay free.

'You were full of consideration – you were offering to make us cups of tea. It wasn't clear if you were being a good host or avoiding lines of assessment. You were very expansive with your body language. What I got from family members was that you were a good communicator, fluent, so the question was, is he more so than normal? I was trying to get a baseline. You gave the impression of not being well, of not being able to keep yourself safe. You were not willing to consider that treatment, medication or admission might be appropriate.

'The doctors then had to consider what they thought would be best. We ruled out the Home-Based Treatment Team. Your family said they were not happy for this to continue and I wasn't sure it would be a safe option, to be fair. I didn't want to put them in a position of having to bother the police again.

'The next option was an informal admission. You were very clear you didn't want it. There are cases when someone will say yes. Some people want to be admitted informally when they know they are ill. There are circumstances when we do that – we try not to use admission, but we will. When you're asking someone to be admitted informally they have to understand that the ward doors will be locked. It's a de facto detention, without giving you the protections of the Mental Health Act. If you're detained, then as soon as you receive the papers you can appeal. Theoretically, an informal admission means you can leave any time, but if the staff decide you're not well enough, that you're not safe, then they have a holding power. Nurses or doctors can stop you leaving and then a Mental Health Act assessment often takes place. But it's difficult to put them in the position of using those powers – if you're sectioned, a consultant is your responsible clinician.'

'So how did it go this time?' I ask Lauren. 'I remember the flat being full of people . . .'

'I was very, very impressed with the police and ambulance crew. The police can put cuffs on – once the paperwork is complete you are liable to be detained. But they were very careful. At this stage I delegate authority to the ambulance crew and police, meaning they get you to hospital. I had several conversations with the hospital – there are guidelines around how you are conveyed: I wrote the report and emailed it to the hospital.

'That's not just the Mental Health Act Code of Practice – these are statutory instruments. I just need to make sure you've got there. I'll often ring family and friends to say they've arrived, they're safe.'

'What did you tell the hospital, may I ask?'

'I said he doesn't have capacity, he's got flights of ideas, his thoughts are all over the place; he's erudite and liable to work his way out of situations, work his way around questions concerning his mental health; he might try to talk his way out of it.'

Lauren and her manager are watching as I write my notes, relaxed but alert. I realise I like Lauren very much. Her defence of eccentricity and her humour seem to underpin the seriousness with which she approaches her work and wields her power. I want to know more about her.

'How often do you get called out?'

'Not every day, then you get three or four the same day. As well as mental health assessments for adults we do cases where there are child protection concerns, emergency mental health work and cases involving homelessness.'

'How do you feel about sectioning people?'

Lauren does not pause.

'The Mental Health Act argues with Human Rights legislation. I'm taking away liberty and rights without going through the Courts from someone who may not be doing anything wrong. It's a huge piece of legislation. Taking rights away from someone when they have capacity is a huge thing. I would be concerned if I didn't feel uneasy about it. We all look back and say, I've detained this many, I've not detained that many, trying to detect any internal bias. You don't do it lightly. We review what we do: what's been the decision-making process? How did we do? I have to be reapproved every five years, and we are all inspected by the Care Quality Commission, who are looking for what happened whenever things went wrong. It's all done in good faith. We just want people to have appropriate support, treatment and care.'

'What do you think of the system?' I ask.

'It does worry me and most health care professionals that people have to travel so far to places where they can be treated. And statistics show admissions are up year on year.'

It suddenly strikes me – her calm and assurance have stopped me seeing it before – that behind Lauren's easy manner and evident pride in her job is a world of witnessed pain.

I ask, 'What's it like to do the job, to section people, to go into those situations?'

'Often I get things when everything else hasn't worked. The decision to detain is often the most straightforward part of it. It's all the things around it that can be complicated. In your case I didn't have to worry about getting the ambulance and police. All these things were ready for me. It gets more difficult if we can't get a bed, if we can't get an ambulance.'

'What would you change, if you could do anything?'

Lauren and her manager exchange glances.

'We are looking for more staff at times of stress,' Lauren says. 'As EDT [Emergency Duty Team] workers we're pretty good at getting the assessment quickly, though out of hours there are only two social workers for the whole borough, covering both adults and children. There are never enough social workers, never enough ambulances. And beds – the Home-Based Treatment Team will call every hospital in the country if they need to, all the way to private providers. I wish there were more therapeutic services, more Home-Based Treatment Teams, more practitioners, more qualified doctors. Lots of people are in crisis. Mental health doesn't exist in isolation; it's the product of a whole set of circumstances. In your case there didn't seem to be stresses in terms of employment. There are people who have no roof over their heads, people who are just getting by. As austerity has bitten we've seen a lot more people in crisis.'

'Are there certain times of year when people are more likely to be in crisis?' I ask.

'We do get a lot of suicides in the spring. It tends to be the liminal times, when seasons change, the big celebrations – Christmas, Eid, football. Football is a nightmare. The World Cup is very busy because of domestic violence, which can lead to child protection issues. Brexit has had an effect. I did one assessment in which their worries about Brexit featured.'

I put it to Lauren that social workers do not enjoy a perfect reputation. In the small and generally well-off town of Hebden Bridge the two cases I know about in which social workers were involved do not reflect well on the profession: one was an adoption which ultimately resulted in an apology from the service involved, the other a bizarre incident in which two off-duty social workers called the police on the mother of a baby who had it with her while she was out drinking a glass of wine.

'Social workers can't just lift children,' Lauren says. 'The police have powers under personal protection orders, Section 20s. But people are scared of us and scared of mental health problems. There's a lot of shame attached to mental health crises – more so in the Asian than in white communities.'

I ask her to tell me more about the different communities she works with.

'Asian families tend to be closer, more interlocked. When we turn up in certain areas it's usually quite obvious who we are and what we are doing. One battered car turns up, that's mine, and two smart ones, that's the doctors, and because it's very obvious quite quickly who we are we do try to keep things very low key. There's an older generation who never ask for help. And under-thirty-fives struggle with everything.'

'How do you approach it then?'

'We try to think about this person's culture, the individuals around them, how the power works. It's about working with people where they are. We look at whether you're using drugs, alcohol, self-medicating if you can't sleep. In your case, when we were told you were a travel writer I determined early on that if you needed formal admission it would be appropriate under our Code of Practice to use Section 2, because that would not stop you doing your job. We were all in agreement. You can be detained for up to six months under Section 3, but because of your job we wouldn't if we could avoid it, because then there are certain countries you can't go to.'

I find myself exclaiming in surprise and something like delight at this. Even before she had met me, while she was establishing what she could about me through conversations on the telephone, Lauren was thinking about the consequences of her possible actions years hence. She seems gratified by my reaction, if surprised that I am surprised to find she thinks and works in this way.

The interview over, her manager clearly satisfied with the way it has gone and her own mind probably partly already on the next thing, Lauren drops her professional guard for a moment. Now she is not a social worker speaking on the record, but someone who knows intimately the worlds and the ways of the maddened. Softly, she says, 'The thread running through it all is holding on to yourself. Illness can be truly horrific. Whatever we do to try to help, we want people to keep hold of the seed, of the thread of who they are, and pull them back.'

I thank Lauren and her manager, and we shake hands. The afternoon is watery with clean, cool sunlight. The two women melt away into streets which are not busy. You would have no idea at all, if you saw them, what hard, strange work they so calmly do.

CHAPTER 31

Self-work

Once a week I go to see my therapist. When we began meeting over a year ago I was incredulous and somewhat wearied to discover that she wanted to talk about my parents, about my childhood. It seemed so clichéd. I wrote a book about them and my upbringing. Wouldn't she rather read that, and save us both a lot of time? She would not. We spent weeks in cerebral battles in which I defended my narrative, while she wanted to know what I really felt, to make me address old feelings in new ways. For many sessions I evaded and dodged her. I had my story of who I was and how I had come to be. I repeated it, shielding my parents from any implied criticism. They are wonderful people who tried hard. My unusual childhood was certainly as magical as it was challenging. Round and round we went. After a long (and expensive) while, everything changed. The breakdown shook my entire self-perception. My understanding of my origins and being seemed to crumble. Coming out of hospital made me different, ready to question, to start again. And I was afraid, in ways I never have been, that if I could not find the keys to fundamental change the madness would come back.

'I don't really think words like bipolar help,' says Jane.

It is not her real name. For professional reasons she asked me to conceal her identity. It feels odd not to be able to name a woman who now knows more about me, in some ways, than anyone ever has. She is about my age, I would guess, with an open face and manner, extremely accomplished in her field, judging by the certificates on her wall, and as deeply sympathetic as you would hope someone in her position would be.

'But you do go up and down. If we can find what is causing you to go high maybe we can stop it, and if you don't go up you won't need to come down. You're never going to be on a straight line – who wants to be? – but the idea is to reduce the amplitude of the ups and downs.'

I press her on her thoughts about bipolar disorder: if I am not suffering from that, or if what I have undergone is better called by another name or understood in a different way, then what is it?

'Have you heard of the Power Threat Meaning Framework?' she asks, and sends me off to read about it.

Researching this term it became immediately clear to me that many psychologists, therapists and growing numbers of psychiatrists believe that the current approach to mental trauma is not working. In 2013 the Division of Clinical Psychologists, under the aegis of the British Psychological Society, published an extraordinary paper which took the view that the current system of classifying and treating mental distress is 'fundamentally flawed'.

The paper took aim at the *DSM*, the overwhelmingly influential *Diagnostic and Statistical Manual of Mental Disorders*, published by the American Psychiatric Association, and at the International Classification of Diseases. These two directories are used to determine whether or not you have a disorder, what it is, and therefore what sets of pills you should take. The clinical psychologists called for a 'paradigm shift' away from these tools – upon which your doctor and psychiatrist will base your diagnosis, should you have a breakdown tomorrow – towards an entirely different approach.

Five years later, in 2018, the psychologists came up with an alternative model, which they named the Power Threat Meaning Framework. The British Psychological Society calls this a 'conceptual alternative' to the way we have been thinking about and treating mental distress. Rather than seeing my case as a straightforward example of an illness which requires medication, the Power Threat Meaning approach places me somewhere on a scale of human experience. There are not, according to this framework, mad people and sane people. I did not cross from well to ill, as the current system has it. Instead, I experienced social, psychological and biological conditions which put me in harm's way. I therefore found myself in need of social, psychological and (to a more limited extent than general psychiatry currently recognises) medicinal help to move back towards the safe end of the scale.

The crucial point is, as the British Psychological Society puts it: '"Abnormal" behaviour and experience exist on a continuum with "normal" behaviours and experience.' Furthermore, 'Experiences and expressions of mental distress are enabled and mediated by, but not in any simplistic sense caused by, our bodies and biology.'

According to this view, my biological triggers and fuels were cannabis, spirits, stress, exhaustion and sleeplessness. The underlying condition which they ignited – a propensity to mania followed by depression – might itself be caused by any number of factors: early trauma, events of childhood and adolescence, certain fixed world views, prejudices, drugs and alcohol, factors in my home and mental environments, guilts, unrealised desires, unfulfilled dreams . . .

As my therapist and many like her point out, science can neither deny or prove that it was these phenomena, rather than something amiss in my brain, that caused me to act as I did. The aim of our sessions is therefore to address early traumas and fixed patterns of belief and behaviour in order to free me from my buried guilts and convictions and their consequences, including drug and alcohol use, which drive me to mania and depression.

Today we are discussing an incident in my childhood.

'Describe it to me. What is happening?' she says.

'We are in the car on the motorway, on the M4. It is the journey we do a lot, driving to Wales on a Friday night. It's dark. My father is driving, my mother is sitting next to him. My brother is very young, maybe four, so I am six. My mother is telling stories; we are coming up to the Severn Bridge, she is talking about the "Pobble Who Has No Toes", the Edward Lear poem. My father is not saying anything. Everything seems to be all right but it isn't. He's often very quiet and my mother talks a lot.'

'How do you feel?'

'Tense.'

'Why?'

'Because my father is not happy and I think it is my fault.'

'Why do you think that?'

'Well I know now that he wasn't happy with my mother, I knew that at the time, but the farm was a disaster, losing money, and he was . . . he must have felt trapped. Every journey up the motorway to this crazy life must have felt mad to him. And if they hadn't had children he would have been free. Dad was very worried and he had problems. He was married four times – my mother was the second.'

'What would you say to that little boy, what would you say to you now, if you could be in the car?'

'I would say, it's OK. It's not your fault. They both love you and it isn't your fault they aren't happy.'

'Go on. Speak to him, speak to that little boy.'

'I would say, "It's really not your fault. The fact is, your dad needs help. He needs therapy. But he loves you very much and you haven't done anything wrong."'

'Yes,' she says. 'Children cannot separate what is happening from the ego – they think everything is about them. So you thought it was your fault. What we want is your mother to stop telling bloody stories and your father to stop being silent. They needed to tell you what was happening, to say, look, adults make mistakes. They get into trouble. It's not your fault.'

Later in the session something wonderful comes.

'We drive on to the bridge in the darkness and there is the sea below, the Bristol Channel, and Dad winds down the windows, he lets all the wind in. And the tension breaks. We are all looking at the sea and it's just . . .'

Suddenly, with clarity and certainty, I realise that it happened then and it kept happening when we were at the farm: when we all looked at the sea, or at our spectacular view of the valley and the mountains from the farm, we were all uplifted; we were together and calm. The tension broke. My parents were moved and soothed by nature in the same way, and I learned this from them. It was always there for us, and we were united in those moments, free from pain and worry. That is what nature has always done for me. It started there. The revelation is so strong I start crying, partly in gratitude for the way the world helped us, the way it has always helped me. For the first time I under-stand that therapy works – actually physically, tangibly works. Breakthrough.

This is the basis of Jane's approach, and now I am convinced by it. Next, using EMDR, we spend hours on another scene. Eye movement desensitisation and reprocessing is a trauma therapy, in which Jane specialises. It is apparently simple. By engaging and distracting the conscious mind, we can access the unconscious, its buried areas of repressed pain and emotion, and by disinterring them and feeling them again, we can free them, and ourselves from them.

In practice this means beginning by holding two vibrating
nodes, palm-sized pieces of plastic, which pulse alternately,
as I recall and re-experience the memories. The idea is that
the vibrations distract my conscious mind, giving me better
access to the unconscious, to buried feelings. Before we start,
Jane asks me where in the body I feel the stress of the scene
– usually in my stomach or chest – and how intense it feels,
on a scale of one to ten.

As we progress, Jane will use the nodes less and utilise
my eye movement to distract me instead, switching her
finger from side to side through the air, while I follow it
with my gaze. Further on still, she will sit very close, move
her finger fast and randomly, and get me to count and tap
out sequences on my thighs and the leg of the chair. Asking
me to enter a traumatic scene from my past, she will push
me right to the point where keeping time, following her
finger and accessing the memories reaches a pitch of intensity
where I can barely keep up. She will make me count the
sequences backwards and in French, pulling my conscious
and unconscious minds apart, and all while asking me to
face feelings from my past, the aim that I experience them
again. The idea seems to be to stop me thinking on one level
entirely, and have me only feel. The latter stages are emotion-
ally overwhelming.

One memory we work on is a summer night at the farm.
My father is not there; he must be in London. It is after
sunset, a dimming green twilight, the valley breathless, the
Brecon Beacons reclining under the sky. My brother and I,
five and seven, are in bed. But something has gone wrong
with the sheep – some ewes or lambs have broken out and
Mum needs to get them back in their fields. She is out there
now, just out of sight behind the trees, a few hundred yards
away, somewhere in the hill fields, but I can't see her.
And now a terrible panic comes over me. I can imagine her
slipping, falling, breaking her leg, unable to make it home.

I start to cry and fret. I run out of the house in my pyjamas crying and shouting.

'What does it feel like? What is going through your mind?' Jane prompts.

'I know that it is probably all right, that she's just there, that she will come back, but I can't help it. I'm screaming and crying because I'm terrified that if she doesn't come back it will be my job to look after my brother and me and I won't be able to do it. And I'm so angry with her, and furious with myself, because I know that by losing it I've let her down – I'm supposed to trust her, support her. This is supposed to be a great adventure, a magical childhood, but because I can't handle it I'm making this crisis, and she'll be angry because she desperately doesn't want us to be worried. And my brother's fine – he's in bed, he can't understand what all the fuss is about.'

'What does it feel like?'

'Shame. Terrible shame. Because I'm in hysterics and I'm shouting – I think I'm shouting any swear word I know. And I'm letting us down . . .'

'Now I want you to imagine you are there, as you, now, looking at the scene. What would you do?'

The perspective changes. Now I am not the small boy; instead I am there, as me, now, physically present in the back garden by the kitchen, watching him screaming and reading his mind. *He will have to look after his younger brother and he doesn't know how he can. He has failed to be who he wants to be, his mother's right-hand man.* (For many years this thought will haunt my mother and me. 'I worried you,' she will say, 'I confided too much in you, I put too much respon-sibility on you.' 'No,' I will say, 'it was wonderful up there. We were fine.')

I am outside the scene but also in it. Jane prompts me and I go to the little boy and pick him up. I hug him and he calms. I nuzzle him foolishly. I point to the field, just there, where his mother is. See? She's safe. She's close. It's all OK. I've got you. You don't have to feel guilty. It's right that you were worried. Any child would be worried. Of course you need your mummy with you, in the house. But you don't have to be frightened. No one is going to leave you. You will always be looked after. We turn and sway. The valley is a music of twilights below us. The far hills dim. I think I make him laugh.

'What did you get?' my therapist asks, meaning what feeling did I get, and where in my body, when I picked him up.

I am crying. 'Calm. In here.'

It is astonishing, that calm. It feels soft and clear, like a silver-blue light, right in my core.

This is a shortened account of a process which took many sessions. Jane helps me to accept that I did nothing wrong, that I should not have been put in that position, that a little child needs his mother in the house, and that, crucially, it is OK to have feelings, to express them and not to hide them, that no shame or guilt need be attached to them. It seems I have spent years, much of my life, concealing many true feelings from myself and others.

We spend weeks on other scenes, especially one in which my brother and I are with my father in a playground in Holland Park one evening after school. Alexander is four and I am six. While he dutifully clambers around on the climbing frame (he is doleful, he knows there is something wrong), my father and I sit on a bench and Dad explains to me that he thinks it will be better for all of us if he and our mother 'don't live under the same roof'.

Though it feels fruitless sometimes, and repetitive at others, the work Jane does with me on this scene changes my life. I experience and understand feelings about my father, my mother and myself I did not know I had.

In summary, it seems that around this time I learned to split myself into an appearance and a reality. In the appearance

I was fine. I was a bright and empathetic child, balanced and well adjusted, an act I have maintained or attempted to throughout my life. But at the same time I was learning to lie to myself and those closest to me. When my father asked me if I understood, I said yes, to please him, to help him, to try to keep him. But I was concealing feelings, fears, needs and realities, becoming accustomed to burying deep doubt and confusion behind a façade of coping. I internalised formidable convictions about my self-worth, about my capacity to understand, to be good, to be loveable. In my heart, it seems, I believed he was leaving because I had failed to please him, to keep him, and because my mother had failed too – she was not good enough. We were not good enough.

Jane takes me through alternative ways it could have gone. Imagine I had said, 'No, I don't understand. Is it because you don't love me? Is it because there's something wrong with Mum?' Imagine my father had said, 'Look, we messed up. This marriage is making me miserable, and your mother. We have made this mess. This is not happening because we do not love you but because I need to get away from your mother to be happy . . . This is happening because adults make mistakes.'

Perhaps then the splitting inside me, dividing what I felt from ways in which I appeared and behaved, would not have been so deep, so long-lasting.

Much later, the pursuit of derangement, distraction, re-assurance and succour through perfectionism; through my versions of the attainment of fortune, glory and recognition; through drugs, alcohol, sex and thrill-seeking became my remedies. And so I went high, and so I went low.

Doggedly, patiently, methodically, Jane helps me to unearth these feelings – I think of them as dirty crystals buried in my core – to hold them up to the light and, by feeling again the feelings that put them there, to smash them.

After every session I tell Rebecca what Jane and I have been working on. Every meeting gives me something to take home. One evening my son and I are playing a form of handball, batting a balloon between us across the dining table. I realise that this is working in an echo of the way EMDR does, distracting our conscious minds, leaving us a relaxed space in which to talk. We are nattering about this or that. I apologise for something, some argument we had earlier, and I say, 'You know, adults make mistakes. We try to be the best people and the best parents we can, but you must understand we're only people, just like you but a bit older. We make mistakes all the time.'

He seems tickled by this. 'Really, Dad?' he says. 'Adults make mistakes?'

'Of course! Everyone does! It's just a question of doing your best . . .'

And I think, is this the time to raise it? To address the breakdown, and why Mummy and Daddy split up for a while? Should we talk about that now? No, I decide. He's easy, he's well and he's fine. There will be plenty of time for that . . . But how useful to know that playing with a ball or a balloon might be the perfect way to talk about serious things.

This is just one of many occasions when something I learn in therapy comes home with me. Having spent a great deal of my life throwing myself into and coping with the consequences of vicious circles, it is quietly amazing to feel that virtuous circles have an equal power, that you can put a life together as firmly as you can throw one away.

At my first appointment with Jane I could not have been more sceptical about the efficacy of psychotherapy, or more ignorant about the processes and results of EMDR. As the journal *Scientific American* put it in 2012,

Few psychological treatments have been as widely heralded as EMDR. Some EMDR proponents have called it a 'miracle

cure' and 'paradigm shift,' and ABC's *20/20* proclaimed it
an 'exciting breakthrough' in the treatment of anxiety. More
than 60,000 clinicians have undergone formal training in
EMDR, and the EMDR International Association (EMDRIA),
a group of mental health professionals dedicated to promoting
the technique, boasts more than 4,000 members. The organisation estimates that this procedure has been administered
to approximately two million clients.

However, the journal goes on to conclude: 'EMDR ameli-
orates symptoms of traumatic anxiety better than doing
nothing and probably better than talking to a supportive
listener. Yet not a shred of good evidence exists that EMDR
is superior to exposure-based treatments that behaviour and
cognitive-behaviour therapists have been administering
routinely for decades.' Paraphrasing Samuel Johnson,
Harvard University psychologist Richard McNally sums up
the case for EMDR nicely: 'What is effective in EMDR is
not new, and what is new is not effective.'

Nevertheless, it is an unequivocal fact that Jane and EMDR
worked for me. Our meetings constituted one of the most
astonishing journeys in a life of travel, and perhaps the most
transforming. There was nothing nebulous or open-ended
about it; we addressed a series of traumas, brought them to
light and, if we did not heal them, we vastly diminished their
power to hurt me, and through me, many others, not least
those closest to me.

Where psychiatry offered me nothing but pills which inflict
proven long-term damage and, while attacking their symptoms, do nothing to address the causes of trauma and
psychosis, psychotherapy changed my life, relatively quickly.
At £60 a session, I estimate I spent less than £2000 on
working with Jane over two years – a lot of money, but a
fraction of what I have blown on drugs, alcohol and the
pursuit of sex.

Around the edges of our sessions we discussed the wider story of treatment for bipolar, and the potential of the Power Threat Meaning Framework to change the conception and treatment of mental distress. The speed and extent to which we steer treatment away from chemical comfort and towards different kinds of therapeutic healing will depend on doctors, NHS decision-makers and politicians, local and national. I next take my enquiries to them.

CHAPTER 32

The people in charge

The chain of authority linking those who care for the severely mentally afflicted begins with the staff on your locked ward. I go back to Wakefield to interview Ben Owens, the nurse who looked after me in hospital. His presence was one of the best things about the ward. He exuded calm and sensitivity, a blend of professional commitment and obvious humanity. You felt reassured that you were in his care. He suggests we meet in the café of Wakefield cathedral.

Ben is tall, gentle, with film-star dark green eyes, full of sympathy and interest. From the Wirral, his accent is soft, lending his voice an edge of quietness. He is in his mid-twenties. Today he looks like a man who has not quite slept off an exhaustion; he is pale, dressed for off duty in a smart Patagonia top.

We sit in the quiet of the café, surrounded by the retired, who give the place an air of slow-moving gentility. I begin by asking how he came to be working here in Wakefield. In one of our conversations on the ward he told me that he had studied at Liverpool John Moores University, where I taught until quite recently. If he had chosen Creative Writing he would have been one of my students.

'I did a mental health nursing degree at LJMU, a three-year course. We did placements at a busy inner-city acute ward, mixed sex, much more chaotic than Wakefield. There are lots of drug-related issues. You get people using crack cocaine and heroin on the wards, females self-harming, it's more frequent in women. There was one who used to blood-let. You responded to an alarm and she would be bleeding herself into an Oasis bottle. She would secrete items to cut herself with. It's quite disturbing to see. I'm a bit squeamish. It's quite traumatic. And there's ligatures – ligatures are endemic throughout acute services. You're always on edge. You go to check on someone and you can't see them – where are they? Are they hanging behind a door? It's a constant anxiety.

'I also did a placement at Ashworth in Liverpool, that's the high-security high-risk ward. Ian Brady's there. It's very restrictive. They say it's harder to get out of Ashworth than it is to get out of prison. There are highly psychotic individuals, people with personality disorders. Some of them will go back to the prison system.'

'Why did you decide to do it, Ben?' I ask.

'I'd had different jobs before but they seemed to naturally build towards nursing. I was a support worker for people with learning disabilities. I was a clerk, ferrying case notes around various hospitals . . . I never had a firm intention, but I have an empathy towards people who are struggling – young lads, they're unemployed, their relationships break down – I empathise. It drives me to listen, to see if there's anything I can do.'

I ask him about his training.

'At LJMU we did anatomy and psychology, general nursing – that's how I met my girlfriend, she's a nurse, working in oncology. That's how I ended up in Yorkshire. We did psychiatric modules, therapy, policy, diagnosis. After the degree you do a four-day course with the NHS trust. You do a lot of role plays; you learn physical restraint and hold-breaking techniques. A lot of treatments are a shot in the dark. If a procedure is effective, we roll with it. It's strange, compared to physical health. Like electro-convulsive therapy – there's no kind of formal neurology, no one knows how it impacts patients, but we've rolled with it. If it's deemed to have a benefit then . . .'

'And then you got your first job?'

'Yeah, Wakefield was my first job. I moved to the area. I felt like a fish out of water. I had impostor syndrome! I'm quite shy. It took a while to adapt.'

'So how does it work? When you were treating me, for example – what do you take into account when you're deciding on treatment?'

'The way it works is Dr X meets with the multi-disciplinary team and we discuss presenting circumstances, what's happened. We feed back observations. We look at historic diagnoses, and Dr X calls the shots.

'If we objected or thought the person was struggling we would put forward that case. It's a collaboration but Dr X has final say. Medication is prescribed. If there's a case for additional medication he prescribes it. The common ones are lorazepam, benzodiazapine, promethazine – that's an anti-histamine but it has a sedative effect. They're prescribed as tablets, but if we feel it's in the person's best interest we can administer with an intra-muscular injection. That's the last resort. We'll say, "Look, a forced injection is not pleasant to do, it's not pleasant to see." There are various protocols. We have a frank discussion – we say, "The intra-muscular will not be comfortable for yourself . . ." It must be awful, I do have a lot of empathy.'

Repeatedly in our conversation Ben comes back to this – to what it must be like to be sectioned, to be locked in, to be forced to take medication, to be injected against your will.

'It must be horrible,' he says several times. 'I can't imagine what that must feel like,' he says.

He looks at me searchingly at these moments and his eyes are haunted. I think he well imagines, possibly too well imagines, given the demands on him, what it is like.

'Can you describe meeting me?'

Ben smiles, takes a breath.

'There's a handover – the day shift give you an overview of all twenty-two patients. It takes about forty-five minutes. It was briefly explained how you'd ended up here, how you were presenting, there was an outline of the incidents. I had to make sure you were aware you were detained. I remember meeting you by the office. I was getting set up for shift. I do remember speaking at one point. You said you wanted to go home. I tried to explain that wasn't happening. It's something I struggle with, these difficult conversations. I remember you were quite frustrated and unhappy about being detained. You were insisting you wanted to leave. I was trying to explain that that was not possible.

'I remember you threatening to call all the newspapers.' He grins. 'And I spoke to you the day after. Everyone's different – it's hard to get to know a person but you seemed quite rational. We make notes every day on how the patient has been, which is relayed to each shift in the handover. And the fundamental point is to make you secure, to make sure knives aren't being secreted on the ward or anything like that, to ensure your safety.'

'How many of the people you treat will be cured?' I ask.

'About a quarter are discharged and relapse, person by person. Having said that, people suffering from first-time psychosis and mood disorders tend to return. Personality and mood disorders are maladaptive: it can be difficult for them to break the cycle. With anxiety and depression, a stay in hospital can solve an immediate problem – it can keep a person and other people safe. It's not great for everyone but it does serve a purpose.'

Nationally, the number of detentions under the Mental Health Act has increased steadily over the last few years. In 2018 the Care Quality Commission revealed an astonishing rise: 'In the ten-year period between 2005/06 and 2015/16, the number of detentions increased by 40 per cent – from 45,484 to 63,622,' it reported. I ask Ben why he thinks that is. Is it rooted in social change? Or is there now a different threshold for treatment?

'I don't think there's a single answer. Our model is based on concern for acute crisis, which we manage with therapeutic treatment and medication. The drive and ethos is empower-ment and autonomy, to keep people out of hospital and in their community. It's about setting someone up to succeed. Of course [illegal] drugs play a big part. But it's chicken and egg – do people do drugs because of mental health problems or do these drugs cause the pathologies? Almost everyone you see has some history with drugs.'

'What would you change, if you had the power to do anything?'

Ben does not hesitate.

'The biggest thing would be the staff–patient ratio. Some days you feel you didn't engage with anyone, you didn't engage with the people enough, which is a great frustration because it's what I went into the job to do. It's almost a cliché in nursing – you don't get enough time to work with people. I had a really good experience recently around the pool table. It's a great leveller, you feel you're all together. But on a busy twelve-hour shift you start, you get no break, you finish the day, that's it. I can't think of another occupa-tion where you might be listening to someone pouring their heart out or dealing with a ligature or a hostage situation. We had one the other day. A patient locked himself and a member of staff in the office. He had broken pool cues he was using as weapons, he used a fire extinguisher to cover up the windows. In the end he called his mum. He was giving the member of staff reassurance all the time . . . I can't think of another occupation like it.'

We talk about workers on the ward we both know; one particularly charismatic man in particular – Hector. It was a conversation with him, when he reassured me that he would be happy to be treated by Dr X (he said he had seen much worse consultants) and intimated that I would be going home at some point, before too long, that made all the difference to my morale and, from that point on, the way I thought about my detention.

'Oh yes, Hector!' Ben's face breaks into a wide smile.

'Health support workers like him are brilliant, respectful people. There's no hierarchy with them, between care giver and care receiver – they break down the barriers. It's different being in the position of nurse – you can stop people leaving; you can detain people for a brief period.'

I ask who looks after Ben's mental health, given the pressures on him and his colleagues.

'We have debriefs with the Management of Aggression and Violence Team – we have input from the ward psychologist. People say if you go into mental health nursing you must expect violence and aggression. After an incident you are offered a debrief. More recently it's been quite difficult. The sense of violence, some of the aggression, when you get a gang of patients who don't click. Staff say that you just need one shift when two people are at home, off sick – there can be just three of us on a night shift. That's really, really low numbers if something were to happen. When you're more experienced you tend to know if something is going to happen. You see things building through the day – you can see someone's mental health declining. We had one the other day someone was self-harming, someone with psychosis was attacking another patient and a group of patients were falling out. It was chaos. We called for staff from other wards. We split them all up. Someone swallowed a bottle top on purpose to self-harm. We did the Heimlich manoeuvre. I think if I was a patient in there then or had a family member in . . . it would be an awful experience . . .'

Ben searches my eyes again. I know I was lucky. I got away with the thin end of the illness. I was sent to a good ward with great care. Thanks to his account I can begin to imagine something of what Ben has seen and dealt with. The cruelty of the dilemma is plain: there is no one you would rather be treated by than Ben Owens, yet the humanity and empathy which make him so good at the job are the very qualities which place such a strain on him. We talk about being the one who has to break the news that you are detained, as in my case. What gets you through?

'The team and the camaraderie. There's a shared sense of humour which gets you through the job and stressful situations. But at the end of the shift you always feel you're leaving people . . . I did four nights in a row, 7 p.m. to 7.45 a.m., and I couldn't sleep, just no sleep at all. I was due on the next day and I got really bad anxiety. I had breathing problems – I thought is it psychological? I had to take a week off sick. Switching from a series of nights to days is not good for your health.'

I have a final question for Ben; he has already given me much longer than the hour of his time I requested. 'Do a lot of us suffer the same delusions? Do you find yourself dealing with the same fantasies?'

'Yes, there are common themes. They're in touch with God or the Devil. Government persecution is a popular one. And being married to Kylie Minogue.'

On the train back to Hebden, I go over and over my notes and everything Ben said. How could we better serve people doing the vital, always stressful, sometimes terrifying job he does? It sounds as though higher staffing levels, more support at work, more humane shift patterns and a system that is better at healing people, rather than simply maintaining them, are the very least we owe him. And he said, 'You don't go into it for the money,' but it is a safe bet he is worth more than he was paid.

Another question lingers as I make my way home. What on earth is it about Kylie Minogue?

My next destination is Halifax, a riddle of a town scattered over the slopes and deeps of a confluence of valleys. A clutch of hills nose together like beasts around a trough. In one tight cleft is Dean Clough, where huge mills have been repurposed into offices, cafés and a hotel. On the fifth floor of one is the headquarters of the Calderdale Clinical Commissioning Group, which dispenses an annual budget of £315 million on behalf of the 215,000 inhabitants of Calderdale. Its chief officer, Dr Matt Walsh, was in touch with me after the broadcast of an essay I wrote about my time on the ward. He invited me to meet him any time, saying in his message that he wanted to show me some of the developments taking place in mental health in our area.

Calderdale makes an acute case study in the ongoing battle for better public health. Rates of depression, suicide and the prescription of antidepressants are very high here. There are pools of long-term unemployment and the lowest levels of social mobility. There are valleys, famously – Hebden is one – where in the winter, in certain places, the sun never shines, shut out by the low brows of the moors.

Of a chief officer wielding a significant slice of the taxpayer's money on behalf of the NHS I was expecting a sharp suit, jargon, a mind accustomed to systems, discourse busy with schemes and undertakings, directives, deliverables and metrics. Matt Walsh is nothing like that. A gentle, sweetly smiling man, he would be your ideal family GP, attentive and compassionate. There is a tirelessness and open-heartedness about him which must make him an inspiring leader. He reminded me of a sea captain, smart and slightly bristly, with that directness which speaks of someone with much to do. Amid the books and pictures of birds in his tiny office there is little sign of what he actually does.

'I'm a GP by background,' he told me. 'I've spent the best part of thirty-five years in health and care, the last fifteen in jobs like this – director jobs across West Yorkshire. The frustration I felt was – we're almost aiming for the wrong things. We're driven to looking at problems rather than lives. Medicine becomes specialised and super-specialised but in the middle of that, lives get lost. We needed to reconnect with the purpose of improving people's lives. Like Active Calderdale – reconnecting people with exercise. We know it's as powerful a drug as you could wish for. It's all about connecting and reconnecting. There are so many forces pulling us apart and we feel a responsibility to push in the opposite direction. It takes courage and a willingness to confront reality. The world is ready for conversations about what a good life looks like, what a good death looks like. I know that my team is able to make a difference. There were cases of young people waiting *two years* to get a diagnosis of autism spectrum disorder. We had a meeting about it and half of us were crying at the end. We've made progress. Over the next twelve months it will be down to eighteen weeks, and I want to get it down to a zero wait-time.

'I want to turn around the commissioning conversation – a change in the relationship between me and my health, realising health is also about states of mind, choices of being, vision, belief, hope, the possibility of joy. It's *these* things that keep us well and happy. So for example we are investing in Improving Access to Psychological Therapies [IAPT] because we realised we needed to start prioritising relation-ships, outcomes, kindness.'

IAPT is designed to combat the shortage of psychother-apists available on the NHS and the gruelling waiting times to see them. You meet a therapist who helps identify your difficulties and suggests coping strategies. Therapists are also available on the phone and at weekends. IAPT aims to provide aid in crisis, short-term therapy, longer-term cognitive behav-ioural therapy (CBT), support for chronic conditions and access to the full range of services the NHS and charity sector

offer. It seems a sensible and practical response, and it is
showing good recovery rates.

'When I was a GP,' Matt says, 'I had a deep frustration
about two things: a willingness on both sides – the doctor
and the patient – to medicalise unhappiness and create
dependency as a result. But people felt they had nowhere
else to go. And a GP wants to help, so you write a prescription. Now we're in a different place. CBT and IAPT have
changed the experiences of some, but we've shifted the bottle-
neck further up the chain. We haven't got enough clinical
psychologists. It's a revealed need, and the need has grown
with austerity, there's no question. The outgoing national
director of public health had it in his report, so did the UN
special rapporteur. It's shameful, the health and psychological
cost of austerity.'

Matt is quick to point out that his own budget was
protected against the cuts, emphasising that the burden has
fallen on other areas of society – education, social care,
policing, local government – which in turn creates an
increased demand for health services.

'We have to think about how we connect people in poverty
to employment – we know wealth drives better outcomes for
care. We need to build capacity in the third sector, in the
arts, in the community. The answers are in *ourselves*, in our
relationships to people. And we need to be clever about where
we go for help. In 1991 when I came into practice there were
about a hundred pathways to care. Now there are about two
and a half thousand. So there are loads of ways of helping
people but no one understands them all, so the default is A
& E. In the future we're going to need to use key workers
and digital technology to provide the best paths through it.
At the same time, we're facing a demographic cliff edge – an
awful lot of GPs are over fifty-five. There's the same cliff
edge in hospital consultants and senior nurses. So we went
to Calderdale College and talked to the students about the

situation. We need to build the capacity to bring people in
. . . and radical politicians are definitely going to be part of
the mix.'

Matt deals with multiple hospitals, specialist care centres
and GP practices, the police, the ambulance service, the local
authority and the council, a myriad of individual agencies and
acronyms. From the quiet but perceptible buzz between the
desks where his team are working you sense that the dynamism
with which he and his people approach their tasks is infectious. In the way that certain schools, certain companies and
institutions make you alert the moment you walk through the
door, you can tell there is something happening here.

At the annual general meeting last year Matt began
proceedings by reading a poem. Now he reads me one of his
own, a joyous portrait of a gannet. I think it is wonderful,
easily publication standard. He looks embarrassed and
delighted. (In fact, he will shortly become a published poet,
with a piece on a swift.)

Grinning, he says, 'I find it starts the conversation in a
different place if you read at the beginning of a meeting. It's
about bringing the whole of your life to it, about helping
people to engage with each other wholeheartedly.' He smiles,
and there's a mixture of self-effacement and pride in it. He
is intensely proud of his team. Their ambition in mental
health is to overhaul the services and quality of life in
Calderdale as a whole. Rather than building more mental
health wards, they are aiming to create a society in which
there is less need for them.

Matt introduces Dr Caroline Taylor, a member of the
group's governing body and their clinical leader on mental
health. Caroline is a strikingly energetic woman of brisk
confidence. She observes you shrewdly and rapidly. She
speaks with speed and humour.

'When I took over I found mental health had been so
neglected for so long. A GP would refer you to a psychiatrist

or prescribe antidepressants – it felt as though those were the only options. A lot of us wanted to send people for counselling. There were a lot of counsellors, but how do we know if they're any good or not? Often it wasn't even recognised that someone was presenting with a mental health issue. And whatever they're presenting with there's likely to be a well-being element.'

Caroline is very funny and adamant about the language.

'You don't have mental health – you have ill health or good health! "Mental health" just turns people off! I prefer "well-being".'

She picks up the story of the situation she inherited.

'It was leading to massive prescriptions of antidepressants and anti-anxiety medication, propanol and beta-blockers. Because I am more experienced than a lot of GPs in this area I have more confidence about taking people off medication. Because I want to change the world and I believe that we *can*! GPs can be too scared to take people off medication.

'Often, it's about helping people to address issues that aren't medical. You can get those people to the right advice and out of our system long before anyone mentions medicine. We give specific information about the people you need to phone. At my practice we employed a young woman, Gemma Watkins, as a work wellness adviser. I gave her a target of getting ten people over fifty who were off work with mental health problems back to work. She did it in no time, completely smashed the target. She was shortlisted for a national award. Often the service people need is *right there*, either publicly funded or in the charity sector, like Healthy Minds [a Calderdale mental health charity], for example.'

'From what you have said,' I ask, 'it sounds as though people are being kept on medication to assuage a doctor's worry about what might happen if they came off it, rather than because they need it?'

'Oh yes,' Caroline says. 'But it's changing. Deprescribing. We can save a lot of money in north Halifax, and use it better . . .'

I leave my meeting with Caroline Taylor and Matt Walsh bouncy with hope and optimism. Where it really matters, where the future is being designed and implemented, we have in Calderdale – and therefore across the country too – creative and original thinkers with the power, some of the funds, all of the vision and the mandate to build a better world.

Matt had suggested I meet Robin Tuddenham, chief executive of Calderdale Council. Matt's dauntlessly patient and efficient PA, Zoe Akesson, set up a meeting. Zoe, like everyone I met at this stage of the investigation, was alert to whatever benefit my work might contribute. I was being swiftly co-opted into the system: I agreed to be a patron of EyUp!, a charity which supports the work at the hospital in Wakefield. We began planning a collaboration with the university where I lecture, which will see writers and poets among my colleagues delivering creative writing classes to patients and staff on the wards. In a mad twist, I was asked to cut the ribbon at my own mental hospital at an event celebrating its £17 million redevelopment.

As I go about my research I bring my findings home and discuss them with Rebecca. We have an evening routine, a little bit of 'Mummy and Daddy time' – obtained by allowing our boy his screen or a playfight with the dog – when we take a glass of wine into the garden or out to the front step. Rebecca is following my progress closely. She feels particularly strongly about the topic and this work, for obvious reasons. When I come home excited about, for example, what Dr Caroline Taylor has said about deprescribing, Rebecca is very wary.

'So you're planning to write a book telling people to come off their pills?'

'Well . . . nothing I've heard or read suggests that pills actually *work*, in the long term.'

'Do you know how much damage that could do?'

'Sure, sure. I'm not going to say, come off, but . . . ask about coming off, demand support in reducing doses – I am going to say that, yes.'

Typically, Rebecca has signed up to the bipolar support page on Facebook. She is a compulsive researcher and driven to help people in trouble. While I can barely scan the page without feeling horror and distress on behalf of those posting on it, Rebecca takes time to answer queries and offer advice and support, particularly to relatives and carers trying to cope with a partner or a relative suffering from mania or hypomania. The debates and discussions we have must be echoed in thousands of homes around the country and across the continent. Every minute of every day someone in trauma is arguing with someone who loves them, both in need of help and support. Although the landscapes of the understanding and approaches to mental health (or societal well-being, as it might better be described) through which I now travelled seemed to burgeon with imagination, vim and possibility, the vision of a bright future asks searching questions of the present.

How long will the country have to endure the present turmoil of mounting numbers in crisis, the over-prescription and mis-prescription of drugs, buoyant suicide rates, shortages of therapists and therapies? What will it take to turn the whole leaking, foundering system around? The people responsible for some of the answers to these questions ought to be in local and national government: leadership is what we pay them for. We grant them power over us in the hope and expectation of vision.

CHAPTER 33

The policymakers

The people of Victorian Halifax knew exactly what they expected of leadership, judging by their town hall. Tens of thousands of them came to see the Prince of Wales, later Edward VII, open it in August 1863, crowding the streets, overflowing specially laid-on trains and enduring downpours of rain that even the *Halifax Courier*, which has reported a few dirty weathers over the centuries, described as ceaseless, a pitiless 'real misery'.

The town hall is modestly magnificent, sandstone, defiantly spired in a northern Italian style and robustly portly on the outside. Within, it erupts with busts, mosaics, coats of arms, marble, stained glass and the Victoria Hall, a splendid and unexpected atrium with glass roof, gallery, balustrade, symbolic carvings and cherubs. This is a fit home for the vigour, pride and grip that was to be expected of those who would have the honour and distinction of serving in it. It was the last design of its architect, Charles Barry, who also designed the Houses of Parliament, and it takes me aback. What a place Halifax was then! What ambitions it held for its future.

The building is strangely quiet. In a shadowed room off the Victoria Hall, Robin Tuddenham is a surprising figure. Zippy, natty, southern, you somehow expect to find him surrounded by teams of developers, ideas people, data architects, software engineers and project leaders. But for all the space and grandeur beyond his door, he is alone. It turns out that the court of people I can half-see around him have been merged and cut and synergised into nothing, leaving him with an extraordinary portfolio of responsibilities.

Robin is in charge of Children's Services, Flooding, Health, Workforce Development and Cohesion, Resilience and Migration (remits that run to the Humber). He also oversees Transport, Town Centre Redevelopment and Housing. He has the wiry frame and balance of his passion, mountaineering, and the kind of sharp suit and bright shirt they would expect, in London, of a man who means business. It is the end of the day and the week. He is tired. I can only imagine how much work he will take home with him. But the speed of his glance and the warmth in his grin suggests this is not someone to be stopped by fatigue.

'Hello! Do come in! Would you like a cup of tea or . . .?'

Robin gives me far more time than I expected or he can have meant to spare. Over the next hour he paints a rapid and astonishing picture of the state of Halifax and Calderdale today. He is trying to make them the best places they can be to live in, he says. That means everything from the built environment to the provision of services.

'The south Pennines – it's the darkness and the light! The people, their resilience . . . My challenge is to employ the power of local government to bring agencies together. The council is the only accountable elected body – it gives us legitimacy and it anchors us. We're the second-largest employer. We create the infrastructure, the built and lived environment of the public realm. At the same time, we're dealing with a 35 per cent cut, that's 1100 fewer staff, and we're trying to do more than ever. Look at what we've done with the Piece Hall, for example – the developments there are the outstanding stars of Northern regeneration. On my second day in the job I had to go to London and fight for it

– an all-day assessment with the Heritage Lottery Fund. It's always touch and go!'

Robin oversaw the final phase of the fabulous Piece Hall redevelopment, a magnificent piazza which includes the Square Chapel Arts Centre, the Orangebox Arts Centre for young people, a bookshop, cafés, bars, a library of which he is rightfully particularly proud – the Piece Hall would be a little jewel in any city in the world. Its beauty and vibrancy transforms the experience of visiting Halifax. Of the other end of the scale, Robin says, frankly, 'We've made the bridge harder to jump off.

'One third of children are not ready for school on their first day. [By this he means they have not reached the developmental stage, the basics of behaviour, attention and comprehension which would allow their teachers to begin educating them.] Childhood obesity is increasing. It's about what comes in versus what we can achieve. The condition of the housing stock is poor – draughty old places. Your most basic need is affordable warmth. Then there are ever more children in care with greater and more complex needs, and over ten years our annual budget has been cut by a hundred million pounds.'

I look at him, at his face. We have all heard figures like this on the radio and read them in the news, massive cuts to council budgets every year. But they mean nothing, really, until you listen to a man who has to implement them, who drives past draughty old houses where parents have no money and children no prospects. His expression is frank and everything about him is doughty: Robin, like Matt, like Caroline, like Ben, will not stop fighting. But it seems savage that we should expect them to do it always on the back foot, always in retreat. *Fund and value these people properly*, I think, *support what they are trying to do and they will change everything.* They will change the world.

Robin explains how he works with the cuts.

'We have had to shift money into those areas of acute need. And you look at all the children in care and think, OK, what can I do? It can be the most basic things. For young people, you've got to have bus services in the evening that can bring them into town to see their mates and get them home, or they're trapped. Then you get the risks and fears about more and more young people self-harming.'

He is too involved in his work, too convinced of the possibilities of the positive and the possible, to be downbeat for long.

'We're trying to support mental health in everything we do. We want to reduce duplication, reduce the number of times someone in trouble has to tell their story – we want clear pathways to care. And we're going to need more people working in it. Who is going to want to work in social care? If you're twenty-four, how can we make you want to work here?

'Look at the history. In the 1820s and 1830s life expectancy was around thirty-six. Then, in Halifax, with the Industrial Revolution, philanthropists and business people come together – they almost create a civic family, like we're trying to create one now. They build everything from hospitals and clean water to environmentally healthy abattoirs, infrastructure, parks, museums – palaces of the people! – libraries, housing plans. The second stage is post-war, Attlee, the investment in local government, the state, the NHS. This is the third moment, everything changing, from the fiscal crisis to the digital space to climate change.'

Robin brings in Iain Baines, head of adult services, who outlines some of their ideas.

'We're looking at personalisation and individual support plans. So you would get a prepaid card and you would use it on what works for you. Whether that's a day centre, or alternative therapies . . . And we're looking at ways of using AI – can we provide tools to help you through crisis? Suppose you're suffering from depression. You could have an app that would wake you up, help you get out of bed, even on your darkest days. It would prompt you to do things that help you, like go out and take exercise, get in touch with people, go to a day centre—'

'AI? An app? Really?'

'Yes!'

It is easy to scoff – it flashes across my mind that the last thing the depressed need is more time with their phones – but then, what would *you* do, gentle reader, gentle voter?

In Robin and Iain we have leaders of vision and skill. But ten years ago the council received £137.7 million per year from central government. This coming year it will get £61.7 million. The year after, in the teeth of the pandemic's recession, who knows? Long before the coronavirus cuts hit, more than half of the power to fill Charles Barry's town hall with public servants, more than half the money Robin Tuddenham and his team could have distributed across their vast slew of responsibilities, had been taken away.

At this rate of subtraction the town hall will be abandoned or derelict within a decade. Perhaps the council will sell it off. It was intended for the people, but if we cannot afford it there is sure to be a developer who can.

The people of Calderdale, the people of the North and the people of Britain want, deserve and pay for ready access to expert professionals, should we run into trouble. What we will get instead, it seems increasingly likely, are messages from a robot through an app.

In London, in Portcullis House, across the road from Charles Barry's Houses of Parliament, I ask an evangelist of austerity and Brexit, Andrea Jenkyns, member of Parliament for Morley and Outwood, West Yorkshire, for her views on what she should do about mental health. Andrea has an interest in the subject. We met at the hospital's ribbon-cutting which formally opened its redevelopment.

She is a small and defiant figure in the crowd of lobbyists, civil servants, advisers and MPs. Andrea lives with streams of abuse from those who disagree with her and the condition of fibromyalgia, which causes her constant pain. From the hard right of the Conservative Party, she is an ardent Brexiteer, one of the first to call for Theresa May's resignation, an opponent of what she calls the 'nanny state' (she campaigned against the tax on sugar) and a fan of austerity.

She listens to you through a palpable filter of calculation, perhaps not an unusual trait in an MP. We come to the fundamentals quickly.

'Pretty well every single person with a knowledge of mental health who I have spoken to has said austerity is one of the causes of the current crisis. Would you disagree?' I ask.

'I would say you have to think about what would have happened if we hadn't had austerity,' Andrea returns. 'If we hadn't had austerity we would be in a much worse situation, so the crisis would be worse.'

'What can politicians do to help the situation – how can you influence policy?'

'Well, for example, you can meet the minister. If you have tea with the minister you can raise issues with them.'

'You can have tea with them?'

'Yes.'

'Are there things that you are particularly interested in, in the field of mental health?'

'I am very interested in how we make the NHS sustainable. I want to get together a committee to discuss the future of the NHS. I don't have the answers but I think it's really important we start working on making the NHS sustainable.'

It strikes me that in order to make the NHS sustainable we would simply fund it properly, and that when she says 'sustainable' she means part-privatised, but I leave it. When we met in Wakefield, Andrea explained that it was her father's treatment at the hands of the NHS which inspired her to enter politics. He died in a Wakefield hospital from MRSA, a death that Andrea felt was preventable and unnecessary, a consequence of poor conditions in the hospital.

'I went into politics to hold the NHS to account,' she said.

We go back and forth on austerity, the need to help people, the importance of treating mental health seriously and supporting improvements in services. We also agree to differ on the consequences of Brexit (Brexit-related depression is widely reported by mental health professionals) because where I see catastrophic consequences for the vulnerable, Andrea sees trade deals and Britain being better off in the long run.

There is an uncomfortable contrast here: Andrea is interested in mental health treatment but wants the state to intervene less in people's lives, not more. Her answer – that tea with the minister is a way in which health policy might change – seemed inadequate and surprising. But it may be the simple truth. Personal chemistry, coinciding or conflicting interests, chance and the strength or otherwise of relationships are precisely the ways in which politics actually functions.

I leave our meeting with the conviction that change, if it comes, will not begin at the top. It is not to denigrate Andrea Jenkyns, whose toughness I admired, to say that she comes from a generation of politicians – my generation, at least in age – who have brought a limited horizon of vision to power. Brexit and reducing the role of the state seem to be their main ideas. Contrast their ambitions to 'get Brexit done' and 'make the NHS sustainable' with the drive and imagination of Aneurin Bevan's generation, for example. The actor and activist Michael Sheen said of Bevan, 'He had a cast-iron integrity and a raging passion.' Meanwhile, a few months after we meet, Andrea Jenkyns will be criticised for receiving a £25,000 salary from a think tank, the Research Institute for Social Mobility and Education, funded by the University of Bolton, that did not then exist. Answering queries by the *Guardian*, as reported by the newspaper in its edition of 5 December 2019, Jenkyns said, 'We have recruited some well-known and respected leaders in the education sector.' A year later, the Research Institute's tangible achievements include a paper and an article dated October 2020 looking at the implications for education and social mobility of the Covid-19 pandemic. The former argues that schools should appoint Virtual Learning Coordinators, the latter that universities should take a blended approach to online and offline learning, an idea which occurred to universities when the outbreak began. A revolution in public health and prospects this is not – or at least, not yet.

Criticisms that politicians are all the same and 'in it for themselves' seem cynical and simplistic, but from an episode like this it is easy to understand why many people think this way. It may be that those in power feel that increasing levels of distress and suffering are unavoidable prices for transforming Britain into a society in which divisions of income and opportunity are ever more pronounced.

While MPs like Jenkyns believe they had perfectly valid reasons for pursuing austerity, there cannot be much doubt about its consequences for the most vulnerable. In 2020 the *New European* newspaper reported, 'last year 92 per cent of NHS mental health trust leaders in England said they believed benefit changes under the Tories have increased the number of people with anxiety and depression'.

Until you look hard at it, the future of mental health seems complicated, depressing and intractable, a societal ill which has worsened steadily and which seems likely to continue to do so. But this is not the case. While it is hard to imagine that radical change in the conception and treatment of mental health will come from members of Parliament, it turns out that the future is being conceived and created in a diaspora of thinkers, campaigners, practitioners and activists in the health service, in voluntary groups and in journalism.

CHAPTER 34

Another way?

An organisation called Compassionate Mental Health is holding a conference in Hereford. Robert Whitaker will be speaking. He is the author of *Mad in America: Bad Science, Bad Medicine, and the Enduring Mistreatment of the Mentally Ill* and its sequel *Anatomy of an Epidemic: Magic Bullets, Psychiatric Drugs, and the Astonishing Rise of Mental Illness in America*. Whitaker is the creator of the Mad in America website, an influential commissioner and publisher of articles critical of drug-based psychiatry. The site also runs courses aimed at care providers and psychiatrists. While his opponents characterise Whitaker as anti-psychiatry, Mad in America rejects the charge. Its mission, it says, 'is to serve as a catalyst for rethinking psychiatric care in the United States (and abroad). We believe that the current drug-based paradigm of care has failed our society, and that scientific research, as well as the lived experience of those who have been diagnosed with a psychiatric disorder, calls for profound change.'

When I read *Anatomy of an Epidemic* I am wholly convinced by its message. The book tells a thoroughly researched and sourced story of an alliance between psychiatrists and drug companies to promulgate the chemical imbalance theory in order to elevate and profit from a treatment model based on psychiatric drugs, which it accuses of doing enormous long-term harm to sufferers of mental disorders of all kinds.

The book causes a deal of ill-feeling at home.

'You read this book and you want to stop taking the pills,' Rebecca cries, 'while I know *dozens* of people who have been saved by taking medication. You don't have a medical background. If you publish a book saying people should stop taking their pills you're going to do damage. And me and the boys aren't going to go through it again. We had an absolutely terrible time when you went mad, and I'm not going to put them through it *any more.*'

Nevertheless, I find the book persuasive and I want to hear Whitaker speak. Although she is understandably suspicious of my interest in the anti-psychiatry movement, Rebecca is wholly supportive of my desire to find out more about it. There is another reason why I am excited about going to the conference, I explain. In the afternoon there will be a session on open dialogue. This is a relatively new treatment and set of beliefs about the entire approach to treatment. It was pioneered in Finland and is reputed to achieve extraordinary results. I cannot wait to find out more about it.

In Hereford we gather in a room overlooking the River Wye. We are sufferers, psychiatrists, nurses, care workers and many parents of the particularly afflicted. The room is sunlit and very calm. The first speaker is Andy Bradley, founder of Frameworks4Change, an organisation devoted to compassionate care. We will each take three cards from the conference, he says, on which are the words 'You matter.' We are to keep one for ourselves, give one to someone close and give one to someone we think may have forgotten.

We are encouraged to talk with the two people sitting next to us about why they came. A nurse and a support worker explain that this is the way forward: talking about mental health not in terms of pathologies, but framing. As Andy

Bradley puts it, 'What matters is the stories we tell. The language we use should not be "I a have mental health problem" but rather "My problems have come from emotional health which has affected my mental health." This makes our story important rather than pathologising.'

Now it is Robert Whitaker's turn. He is gentle with the space he occupies, observant and quiet. His theme is 'changing the script'.

> Changing the script is the big challenge. What we have is not a medical model, it's a disease model. We have to look at what it's wrought and change the narrative. That is the biggest thing – societies and individuals organise around narrative. What we're involved in is changing that narrative of what happens to people, and what are the possibilities.
>
> The story of how we got here has two parts. Drugs called antipsychotics were developed and used in asylum medicine from around 1975. Then in 1980 we get *DSM 3* [the third edition of the *Diagnostic and Statistical Manual of Mental Disorders*, effectively a treatment handbook in which a clinician could look up your symptoms, identify your condition and select from recommended drugs; the manual is now in its fifth edition], which is incredibly powerful. Its ideology was exported around the world. Where did *DSM 3* come from? From the American Psychiatric Association. The guild felt threatened by a rising psychiatry survivor movement, which was like the Civil Rights movement. There was a sense that psychiatry was in competition with social workers and counsellors. Ken Kesey's *One Flew Over the Cuckoo's Nest* was hugely influential. And there was a famous article about psychologists going into hospital, pretending to be mad [This was the Rosenhan experiment, which concluded there was no way of distinguishing the sane from the insane in a psychiatric ward. It has since been investigated by the writer Susannah Calahan, who told the *New York Times* it 'exposed

something real' despite manipulating its results.] So the American Psychiatric Association decided to reform [the] *Diagnostic and Statistical Manual*.

There were other problems too – diazepam was beginning to be seen as an addictive drug. How could psychiatrists restore their credibility, their place in society? They looked at the white-coat approach to infectious diseases. You trust the person in the white coat that you have a disease and they can cure it. So we need a white coat. But how? The answer was, conceptualise depression, anxiety and distress as *diseases*. They restore legitimacy and power to the profession by calling things diseases. This was not a medical model, it was a disease model.

So *DSM 3* makes all kinds of emotional matters, misgivings and difficulties diseases of the brain. This elevates psychiatry: as we call them brain diseases we need a diagnosis for everybody who comes to us. So there is a shift in the conception of normal problems of living. In fact, life is episodic. Anxiety is normal. Psychosis is a failure to adjust to whatever pressures are on you. But now we want diagnosis for everybody; we call them diseases of the brain. This is a *huge* shift. Now we have a line between normal and abnormal. When we talk about changing the script that's the first thing – erasing that line.

In order to support the disease model, psychiatry looked at the brain, at serotonin and dopamine. The stress is now in [the] individual's head – it's not exterior, it's not circumstances – now *you're* defective. And so you get the chemical imbalance theory, which tells of great medical progress. It told the world they had identified the very molecules that cause depression and madness – serotonin. If it were true then it would have been the greatest discovery in the history of medicine.

Who is really happy now? The drug industry. They can't sell you drugs for unhappiness or divorce, but they can get approval for drugs to treat depression. Money floods from industry to APA, to academic psychiatrists – the drug industry effectively buys American psychiatry to seal this story. They build markets. Look at the incredible expansion of the bipolar market, the ADHD market. Now, today, we have juvenile bipolar.

My father fought in Italy in World War II. When he came back he had a breakdown in the US. Dad spent six months in a mental hospital under a totally different conception from what we have today. He had a degree, he was good at his work, he was an accountant – they said you'll be back, your seat will be available. It was understood he had a nervous *breakdown* – he was not diseased, he had had an episode. He went back to work the rest of his life. The whole idea of genetic heredity and predisposition is a huge shift. The drug industry is very successful at building markets.

In 1987 comes Prozac. Now you're looking at a $40 billion market. Twenty-five per cent of kids going to university as freshmen are given a diagnosis and a drug. When Prozac first took hold there was a lot of resistance, especially in Europe. But we exported it around the world – the serotonin definition of depression, including as a treatment for ADHD. Is it true?

In fact, by 1984 it was clear that depression is not caused by damage to the dopamine system. There is no lesion in the brain, no injury in the dopamine system of a depressed person. The APA investigated the dopamine hypothesis and found it was not true. The marketing story had been pitched to the public as scientific but in fact there was no science behind it. But the drugs really do change brain processes.

Drugs block transmission between receptors; drugs act as accelerators; drugs create the abnormality they were hypothesised to solve in the first place. Of course, we might want to use them temporarily, as long as we have a model to get people off them. But here's the thing – treatments should lessen the burden if the disease model works. You would expect that if you compared the treated and untreated then the treated should do better. I looked at the evidence for this form of care.

Recovery rates for schizophrenia are 6 per cent – the lowest it has ever been. For people with a psychosis diagnosis, six or seven long-term studies say the unmedicated have better results. We have switched depression from an episodic anxiety to a chronic disorder. If you look at disability numbers in the US – people receiving disability payments for mental health reasons – in 1987 it was 1.1 million, it's now 5 million. With children, 16,000 families in 1987 have become 700,000– 800,000, two thirds of whom go on to adult disability. We have created a new career track – lifelong mental patients. When *Anatomy of an Epidemic* first came out [in 2010] I said I was looking at the US. Every country I have studied since that has adopted our model has seen its disability rates go up.

Since 1980 we have organised and internalised our thinking about this and the provision of services around chemical imbalances in the brain. It's a failure scientifically. There is a huge failure of outcomes. It has done huge damage to societal thinking. It is a false philosophy of being, that the problem is in the individual. The problem is societies. To suffer is to be human.

We applaud and break for lunch, stimulated and thoughtful. Conversations over lunch are harrowing. Parents, sisters, patients and mothers of patients tell the same story. Up and down the country, round and round the health services, in and out of queues and waiting rooms they have been, trying to get help for a child, a sibling or themselves.

The commonest story is cannabis – skunk – when young, breakdown, and then . . . 'They put my son on a cocktail of drugs. We travelled the country, moving house to find a doctor who would help. And it's, "Let them eat Prozac . . ."'

No one here disputes Whitaker's narrative, though it could be argued that because conventional treatment has not worked for them or their relatives their perspectives are skewed. Talking to the delegates here – the mothers, the former sufferers, the nurses and psychotherapists – I find it hard to believe that they could be convicted of unjustly blaming physicians for the illnessses they have experienced or witnessed. When I first heard Whitaker's story – his talk is a summary of the argument he makes in *Anatomy of an Epidemic* – I was horrified and enraged. It seemed to me that I and millions of other people suffering from similar afflictions, and our families, were being routinely mistreated, paying victims of a cynical system designed to enhance the standing of psychiatrists and enrich drug manufacturers.

But the accusation of conspiracy makes me uncomfortable; rather, it seems to be a case of each element in the system doing only what it does, with the results of their efforts being short-term benefit at best, harm at worst. Psychiatrists would prescribe the perfect drugs, if they had them, and drug companies would provide them if they knew how to make them. The mighty marketing departments of the pharmaceutical world propagate the chemical imbalance theory because it is easy to sell and appears to make sense.

It now seems to me that we are all living with the consequences of nearly a century of a deeply imperfect and extraordinarily profitable system which is clearly in urgent need of reform. But how shall we replace the pills?

Investigating my predicament, I read hundreds of thousands of words in research papers, scholarly articles, journals, magazines, newspapers and books. I was seeking to understand what we know about the causes and treatments of mental disorder, and I was looking for non-drug-based treatments – for a third way between pills and praying. Open dialogue treatment for breakdown and acute crisis stood out to me for two reasons: it involves psychiatric drugs only as a last resort and for the shortest possible time, and it reports stunning results, up to ten times better than those of conventional, drug-based psychiatry.

After lunch, the session on open dialogue takes place in a quiet function room with wooden floors and benches. Most of those attending are women. The speaker is Yasmin Ishaq, service lead at the Kent Open Dialogue Service. She is a balanced presence. Her face is gentle and smooth but for flares of lines at the corners of her eyes.

Her first slide tells the story of two groups of patients treated in Kemi-Tornio, Finland, where open dialogue was developed.

After two years, 14 of the OD group had required bed nights in hospital, compared to 117 of those in the standard cohort. One in three of the OD group had been treated with antipsychotics, compared to all those in the standard cohort. While 24 per cent of the OD cohort had had a relapse, it was 71 per cent of the standard group. Some 81 per cent of the OD group had returned to work, compared to 43 per cent of the standard cohort. (These are the five-year follow-up results, published in 2006).

Comparing the results of the Kent trial which Yasmin Ishaq directs, with identical sample groups from two adjacent areas, Canterbury and Maidstone, the picture becomes astonishing. Urgent referrals to hospital: 82 from the OD programme, against 498 and 702. Thirty-four bed-days for OD, against 2763 in Canterbury and 3027 in Maidstone. The average number of bed days per referral is the number that really hit me, thinking of my time in hospital: 0.5, half a day on average for OD, against 5.5 and 4.7. The OD group were in and out, effectively. The average cost of a bed-day is £390, so the OD programme cost on average £195, compared to £2145 in Canterbury and £1677 in Maidstone.

There are shakes of heads in the room as I marvel at this last statistic. Cost is the last place we should look, the feeling runs. However, we all know that in the age of austerity (and now, in the pandemic recession) nothing beats the bottom line. How on earth do open dialogue, Yasmin and her team do it? She describes the process.

Clinicians working in pairs see the family and person in trouble together. We find words to describe what is happening. In a crisis the family are desperate. They fill in the full picture. Patients and families talk about these first open dialogue sessions as incredible. They say they are fully listened to. The flexibility is key. Sessions can run on, they take as long as they take. At the same time, patients and families don't need to hold on to the crisis longer than they are able to. The patient dictates when we meet again. One of our patients' mothers talked of sectioning – new crisis teams – constant change of people – disengagement by the patient – new crisis. In our model, the clinician takes responsibility for involving other services. It's not the patient or the carer's responsibility.

The clinician makes sure the story evolves from everyone together: I'm not a visitor or someone in authority asking for your history; I'm helping us develop our relationships, building a safer feeling.

Then, we work with uncertainty. We're not making hasty decisions. We own our worries about the risks. We share them with the family and the patient. We sit with our distress, not jumping to quick solutions. We have an open system which means we have to accept and embrace uncertainty. What can we do to help this person maintain the agency of self? We see them as a human being with a vivid experience. We don't label them. We hold our anxiety as a team, as a network.

We try to hear what is said, seen, felt. We give people space to explore. What happens? What makes this person feel bad? What are the causal difficulties? We raise differences of opinion in front of the family.

If the doctor is worried about something they share it,
and we have that discussion there and then. It's about holding
the emotional burden without trying to fix it. We don't always
know whose burden we're carrying. Theirs? Ours? We hold
it as a team. We try to use our knowledge and skills in a
light, gentle way. The emotional burden on my staff is often
greater, but it's how you hold that burden. A lot of it is
scheduling, keeping diaries flexible, it's incredibly challenging. But we have a 2 per cent sickness rate on my team,
compared to 5 per cent in the service.

All the staff are trained in a range of psychological skills
with elements of social network, systemic and family therapy
at its core. The conversation is a frame for families and
patients to increase the sense of agency in their own lives.

We're trying to lower the clinical gaze. To offer help in
ways people can say no to. There are myriad ways of understanding what's going on. There isn't one truth. It can be a
great relief for psychiatrists. They can come to the meeting
without being responsible for having to have all the answers,
without concealing their worries. It's OK not to be sure. The
team psychiatrist dispenses significantly fewer drugs. GPs
want to be part of the conversation. We can and do hold
open dialogue meetings in their fifteen-minute slot.

Yasmin invites questions.

'How do we get your service?' asks one of us.

'A Glasgow man said he would move to Faversham. He was
in desperate need and things were moving too slowly. But
you'd have to meet the criteria, be living in the right GP
cluster, and then be selected for randomised control trial . . .'

A delegate speaks: 'They're not interested in people's
context or history at all.'

The group concurs immediately.

'Diagnosis ends curiosity in the system,' Yasmin agrees.
(I understand her to mean that once you are given a diagnosis

of bipolar, for example, our system has no further interest in the causes, specifics and nuances of your case. That was exactly my experience: following in the tradition of the *Diagnostic and Statistical Manual*, I was given a label and advised to take drugs.)

Although there is raw and traumatised feeling in the room about the standard approach, Yasmin and the audience seem to feel more pain and regret than resentment towards it. Parts of the psychiatric establishment are right with her: her group of eight won the Royal College of Psychiatrists Team of the Year.

Of all the many heroic people I meet in the course of this journey, the one most comfortable with madness and most optimistic about its treatment is Yasmin Ishaq. Some weeks after the conference in Hereford I interview her over the phone, calling her from the flat, where the ceiling by the map room has yet to be repaired. I ask how she came to open dialogue.

'I've been a social worker for over thirty years, a psychologist for five years now. I've been working in mental health services since 1996. In 2011 I heard Jaakko Seikkula [a pioneer of open dialogue] speak at a conference. When I heard him I thought that is *it*! *That* is how I want to work. I spent the next few years researching it, and in 2014 I was contacted by a group of clinicians and researchers and that progressed to a National Institute for Health Research grant, a very large grant, £2.4 million, one of the largest grants ever given out for medical research that is not drugs related.

'In 2014–15 a group of us did a year-long training programme in Birmingham in peer-supported open dialogue. This includes the users' voices, a peer worker who has had experience of mental health difficulties – someone who knows what it's like to be in hospital, to be sectioned, someone with a wealth of experience, which is absolutely invaluable, especially when you are dealing with someone who has been sectioned, someone who has been in hospital, someone who has been forced to have treatment.

'Half of the training is in the network of relationships, half is self-work. You start to understand that those who become well are on a continuum with those who don't.'

It all sounds very good, very kind and accepting, but I try to picture how I would have reacted to a process like this when I was engaged to Kylie Minogue, trying to save the world and under heavy surveillance by multiple intelligence agencies.

'So if I come to you and I am delusional, I have a whole series of fantasies, I'm not connected with reality at all – what do you do?'

'I might say, "I can feel how that distresses you." I'm not going to say you are delusional; I say, "What's that like? Tell us what has happened." It might be family breakdown, something in your childhood, job loss, bullying . . . The moment we get a story it's very easy to say, "That's very understandable. From what you're telling me about what you've been through, what you're feeling is a very normal experience." We normalise it. It's more about healing than curing.'

The distinction has escaped me throughout this story. Of *course*. I have been battering my head against this. I cannot be cured. *There is no cure.* So I am consumed by the fear – upon which I can hardly bear to look – that I will do more damage and be found out, diagnosed as mad again, because I will never be cured. I exclaim, 'Healing rather than curing! That's fascinating!'

Yasmin's voice changes slightly. She seems to come closer.

'Yes. The language we use is very powerful. We're very careful. Someone might come in and say, "I want a diagnosis." The doctors on our team are trained to be very tentative. They might say, "It *could* be this? Or it could be that?" We always work from a tentative position. It's very easy to want to stop the delusions because it is distressing to be with. But we can sit with the distress, overcome the urge to move away. Often that urge is to make *me* feel better. Doctors and psychiatrists, all of us, do things to alleviate our own distress, because our triggers have been hit. So you have to attend to your own experience. Answers do emerge. Meds can help and they can make things go away very quickly, but they hide the cause.'

'So if I come to you and say I think I'm bipolar, I don't want to take this medication, what do you do?'

'I'd say tell me more. "What makes you think that?" Rather than a checklist I want to hear what you are experiencing. With bipolar there's a lot of self-diagnosis; people are always in search of answers. So I'd say, "Let's think about that. Let's invite your friends and family in." Other voices come in and contribute. We want to normalise the experiences behind what you are all going through. Bipolar is a very popular self-diagnosis. But actually, people have different rhythms of emotional regulation. I don't care if they've had a formal diagnosis. I'm more interested in the story behind what's happening. And if I think there is a risk of something catastrophic I will be honest. It's all about being transparent. If I'm worried you might need to be admitted I'm going to say, "I'm carrying this worry," and I will discuss it with other members of the network. We will have that conversation in the room at that moment.'

As Yasmin speaks, all I can see is Rebecca's face, her expressions on all the evenings we have been spending together when she has described what she went through. I think of the desperation and anxiety in her eyes as she thinks that I am going to come off the pills she believes are keeping me sane, the frustration that overcomes her when she thinks about what she considers entirely inadequate support for me from Andrew and the Home-Based Treatment Team, their readiness to tick me off as stable and medicated, and move on. I think about the hopeless obduracy of Dr Y, as I experienced it, as he told me to take lithium and moved on to his next case, his next prescription.

'How does what you are doing go down with the profession?' I ask.

Yasmin says, 'When I talk to psychiatrists I cite Joanna Moncrieff, a psychiatrist they respect. Her point is that when we medicate people we create a chemical change which might be helpful but it's not correcting. The problems are masked. We're treating distress, that's unarguable, but drugs are creating a chemical imbalance. The disease model leads to a prescription of meds which have side effects that touch everything – relationships, functioning. They work as a blunt instrument. Jo Moncrieff advocates the use of these treatments only very carefully. They can be helpful in the short term to manage very high levels of distress. I was on a mental health tribunal and the doctor on the panel said, "Do you think this person should be on a depot [an intra-muscular injection of antipsychotics that effectively enforces compliance] when they are discharged?"

'I said, "They should take their medication in the way they want to take it. If they want to stop they should work with us and we should help them to come off it."

'But you know, just coming off would make them non-compliant. I *hate* that phrase, non-compliant. It takes away all choices and decisions. In our programme, if they want to stop meds, we get the doctor in. We never say, "You need to stay on medication." We say, "If you want to stop then take this level, really carefully, safely, then we'll see." Then we'll check in. Then we'll see if we can reduce it more. It has to be the individual's choice. Doctors are very anxious – they're carrying it. How will this be seen outside? Will they have to end up answering for it in the coroner's court? That drives their risks and worries. I've been in a coroner's court and had to explain decisions. This is a new model. We've lost one in three years. Compared to other areas it's a much better rate. We listen to people and intervene. If someone needs to meet the next day, we'll meet that need.'

I think about my decision to lie to Rebecca about my medication. If we had been in open dialogue, I believe we would have found it easier to talk about me taking the minimum dose of aripiprazole or tapering the drug, and Rebecca would have been vastly relieved of the responsibility. Or we might have maintained our positions and split up. Either way we would both have had support. The mountain of stress and worry we have carried and internalised would have been taken away.

I tell Yasmin, 'I've stopped taking the aripiprazole and I'm lying about it.'

'It's very common,' she says. 'In open dialogue people make decisions about not taking it because they have a space. We review it: "Is it helping? Do you want to come off? Do you need help? It's absolutely your choice." It's not for us to decide.'

I ask, 'Do you think it's going to work? Do you think we're going to see open dialogue become available to people who want it?'

She pauses. 'I don't know. I don't know,' she says. For the first time she sounds tired. 'It would take a paradigm shift.'

Yasmin uses the words softly, as if she fears scaring them off. Beyond my window gathers another Hebden dusk. When she next speaks you can hear something unconquerable coming back to her.

'The next stage is a very large trial – 650 people – then there will be a two-year follow-up, reporting in 2022, 2023. If we can get into the NICE guidelines, *that* will make the difference. We have the top professors in the country, and the leads are the top researchers, hugely respected. Professor Steve Piling at UCL is the lead researcher for the whole programme. It's taking place in Kent, in north-east London,

south Essex, Camden, Islington, Haringey, Buckinghamshire
and Devon.'

'It's good news for southerners, then!'

'They tried to get the North on board too. But they didn't
want it. And there's a chorus in Kent: "We want it in
Medway! We want it in Dartford!" More people are saying,
"Why is it not taken up more broadly?" The hope is for
people – it will change how people are treated in hospital.
The way people are treated now can be shocking. The
language: "They're not compliant; they haven't got insight."
Who are we to say people who have psychosis don't have
insight? They have insight; we just don't have a language
that allows them to share it. Our language is insufficient. It's
up to *us* to find a common insight.'

CHAPTER 35

Full circle

In the autumn of the year which began with my detention and later release from hospital my father died. One of his last requests to Rebecca, whom he adored, was that she ensured I continued to take my pills, the aripiprazole I had long since stopped taking. He never asked me if I was still on them. He rarely told his children what we should do; he preferred to treat us as he found us, and to withhold judgement except in times of crisis. This is the first book I have written that he will not be among the first to read. He was a truly great journalist and an enquiring, rigorous thinker of whom it was once said that he was never professionally happier than when pointing out that the emperor had no clothes. Although he would have been strongly opposed to my decision to come off the pills – particularly as I made it, initially, primarily on instinct – I have tried to follow the art I so admired in him and partly learned from him, of seeking to discover the truth by reading, by talking to people and by recording clearly what I learned. Although it is dedicated to Rebecca, this book is meant as a tribute to him.

When he died in September I had been well since April. The period leading up to his death was calm and full of love, and though his dying was terrible, he left me and all of us in the best way he could, having decided to stop treatment when it was clear that nothing more could be done to help him.

Although I was sane and functioning and able to do every-thing I would have wished to do for him and for those who loved him, I had not completed my course of eye movement desensitisation and reprocessing with Jane. I was still in a raw and shaky place, sliding and unsure-footed on the continuum between sanity and instability, and had not resolved the complications of my relationship with Rebecca (brought about by my behaviour and by what she now knew of the ways in which I had secretly behaved over the years). I was also still lying to her about taking the pills.

In the aftermath of my father's death we hit another crisis. I slept with someone else. I confessed that I had not been taking the pills. I promised to try them. I took them for a few days, over a long weekend when I was performing at a literary festival in Dorset. They made me feel numb, dopey, woozy and disconnected. I felt as though I was stoned. I threw them away, resolved that I was done with them for ever.

Rebecca's conditions remained the same. We loved each other and wanted to be together, for ourselves and for the boys, but unless I took my medication she wanted me to leave. We needed relationship counselling too, to see if there was a way forward for us, to allow us to confront the causes and costs of my behaviour and infidelities. Night after night we faced where we were, where I had brought us to. In pain and fury Rebecca poured out her hurt and her anger. It was no substitute for relationship counselling (we were on private-sector waiting lists, but no counsellor was available) but it was something. She could vent and express her feelings, and I was able to confront, recognise and take responsibility for the things I had done and the places to which I had brought us. Meanwhile, in the sessions with my therapist, Jane and I dealt extensively with the causes and processes of my behav-iour and their consequences in guilt and shame.

Nevertheless, Rebecca and I enjoyed each other's company more and more. I found writing parts of this book horribly gruelling – I will always struggle to read the first half, up to my detention in hospital – but also cathartic and, as it progressed, liberating.

I continued to pretend to take the pills. With every passing week and month, with no sign of mania or depression returning, my decision seemed to me more justified. When finally I did admit the truth again to Rebecca, I hoped she would at least be glad that I had been spared taking thousands of harmful milligrams of harmful chemicals I did not need. The more I researched the outcomes for those taking anti-psychotics or lithium after breakdown, the more thankful I became that I had resisted the drugs.

It was fortunate I did not follow Dr Y's lithium treatment plan, if only because I would have inevitably attempted to come off it. I did not know, when I refused it, that the prescription of lithium, though it has shown to be effective in the short term, dramatically worsens your prospects of recovery overall. Studies have shown that people who stop taking it (around half of all users) are significantly worse off than those who have never taken it: they are more debilitated and less able to live a normal life. Periods of sanity between manias are seven times shorter than if they had never taken the drug. 'Rapid cycling' shifts them from depressed to manic in a matter of days, even hours. Many suffer 'mixed states', a particular hell in which you are manic and depressed at the same time.

Lithium should have been nailed in 1996 in the wake of a study by Martin Harrow and Joseph Goldberg of the University of Illinois which found that after four and a half years manic-depressive patients on lithium fared no better than unmedicated patients. Researchers at the University of California looked at five-year outcomes and came to the same conclusions. Psychiatry has responded to the problems with lithium treatment not by withdrawing it, but rather by prescribing it alongside other drugs.

Professor Joanna Moncrieff summed up the debate around lithium in response to a 2015 article by Jamie Lowe in the *New York Times* entitled 'I don't believe in God, but I believe in lithium'. In her article, Jamie Lowe detailed her manic depression and a twenty-year course of lithium which destroyed one of her kidneys, necessitating a transplant. In response to Lowe's passionate advocacy of lithium, Moncrieff published an essay on her website, (joannamoncreiff.com, 1 July 2015) entitled 'Reasons not to believe in lithium', in which she reviews various studies and trials of lithium. She concludes that no one has ever demonstrated that people who take drugs for manic depression do better than those who do not. 'In fact, overall,' she writes, 'they seem to do slightly worse.'

Moncreiff goes on to say she understands that manic depression is terrifying, and that patients and doctors under-standably feel that there must be something that can help. 'If not lithium, then what?' Moncreiff imagines them asking. She argues that doctors should help people who want to try antipsychotics or anticonvulsants to take them 'as safely as possible, at as low a dosage as possible.' Then she writes, 'But doctors should be honest about the state of the evidence and for lithium, I am not convinced there are any circumstances that justify the risk it entails. In 1957 a pharmacologist bemoaned the fashion for treatment "by lithium poisoning". One day, I believe, we will wake up and realise his concern was spot on!'

Whatever you think of Joanna Moncrieff and Robert Whitaker and those like them who wish to see a radical overhaul of psychiatry and drastic reductions in the prescrip-tion of drugs, the evidence their movement cites is urgently thought-provoking.

One of the longer-term and more respected studies into the medicalisation of mental illness was run by Martin Harrow, who published his results in issue 195 of the *Journal of Nervous and Mental Diseases* in 2007. It would seem to torpedo the entire approach of those psychiatrists whose sole treatment is the prescription of long courses of pills. Harrow's study shows that, over time, manic-depressive/bipolar patients on medication do significantly worse than those off medication. On a seven-point scale, where 1 is normal and 7 severely ill, those who took what the psychiatrists told them to take averaged 5.5 points after two years, while those who took nothing averaged 4 in the same time. After fifteen years, the medicated group were at 5 points, while the non-medicated had sunk to 2. They had taken nothing, so they had no side effects, and they were nearing full recovery.

Deprescribing is taking wider hold. The medical profession has become wary of polypharmacy, the condition in which a patient is prescribed drugs upon drugs, so that some may bolster the effects or counteract the side effects of others. The term 'deprescribing' first appeared in the field of geriatric medication, referring to the reduction or cessation of medication in cases where risks outweigh benefits. The same approach is now growing in the treatment of mental health. As clinical commissioning leaders like Caroline Taylor, psychiatrists like Peter Macrae and GPs in a constellation of practices look at ways of taking people off pills or reducing doses and ranges of medication, deprescribing is becoming part of the professional conversation around the direction of mental health treatment.

In 2019 Swapnil Gupta and John Cahill, both practising psychiatrists who make use of medication in their treatments, and Rebecca Miller, a psychologist, published the first book on the subject, *Deprescribing in Psychiatry*. The authors are adamant that deprescribing should not be thought of as a movement or a fad; rather, they say, their book aims to offer a pragmatic starting point for open conversations between prescriber, patient, clinical team, friends and family in the hope of supporting the decrease of doses or the cessation of medication through a process of shared decision-making. This careful approach notwithstanding, Gupta, Cahill and Miller begin their book with an epigraph taken from a speech given in 2004 by Patricia Deegan, a psychologist and researcher who experienced schizophrenia and then became an activist for disability rights. The passage is a ferociously assertive reminder of what is at stake – the living hell of over-medication.

> We know what it means to be in a chemical tomb, where we feel so drugged we are neither alive nor dead; when we are so drugged that our bodies are stiff and slow and lifeless; when our faces become expressionless masks; when our eyes stop dancing and, instead, glaze over into a petrified stare; when our passion is neutered under powerful pharmaceuticals; and when we are, quite literally, disappeared within a chemical coma.

I have no experience of this kind of entombment, but I have seen people enduring versions of it in hospital, and spoken to people who have been through it. There could be no more urgent argument for new approaches to the treatment of acute disorder, or for a greater role for therapies involving nature, exercise, mindfulness, art, creativity and horticulture, conversations with therapists, and treatments like open dialogue and EMDR.

It is my hope and conviction that in the coming years we will understand and treat mental illness – perhaps we will soon simply call it well-being – in ways we are just starting to try out. I cannot believe that the effective and cost-effective practice of open dialogue will not be hugely expanded, reducing the need for drugs. An arresting figure produced by *The Oxford Textbook of Nature and Public Health* estimates that for every pound the NHS spends on gardens and gardening therapies, five could be saved through reduced care costs.

By December Rebecca and I and our family are in a good way. We decide to go back to the Val di Fassa in the Dolomites. Sparing the staff of the Hotel Medil a reacquaintance with their most chaotic guest of the year before, we book with the same tour company but into a different establishment, the Hotel Dolomitti. At the airport we are met by the same driver, Alex, who picked us up a year ago.

'Looking a lot more sane than you were last year, Horace,' Robin says mildly as we head for the minibus under the same bright sky, the same mountains rearing over Innsbruck airport.

'This time last year I was convinced you were working for GCHQ,' I mutter.

We go over the same pass, through the same dazzle of snow, marvelling at the glittering frozen violence of the peaks and the glowing snowy depths of the pine woods. Our son is jumping with excitement again and Rebecca is lit up. She loves the mountains above all landscapes and has long dreamed of moving us to a chalet in the Alps, where we would keep a cow.

When he drops us at the Hotel Dolomitti, Alex, who recognised us and me immediately, shakes my hand. 'Enjoy your holiday,' he says slowly, looking into my eyes with a kind and serious smile.

We do. Our little boy is a tremendous skier, at six. Robin has mastered black runs. Rebecca is confident on red. On the first two mornings I write while they head for the slopes. I go back to a bar in Canazei where I was certainly mad but where I managed to conceal it. The same woman, Paola, whom I believed last time to be a member of an Italian parachute unit, makes me an espresso macchiato. She recognises me. She seems pleased.

'Ciao! Come va?'

'Bene, grazie. E lei?'

'Multo bene,' she says.

I decide to leave the retracing of last year's exploits there, and instead to learn to ski. I love it. What an idiot I was, as well as a madman, not to have done this last year; what a mad prejudiced, drunken, druggy fool.

'If you get into trouble, Daddy,' the youngest advises, 'just go *faster*, like this!'

We ski together. At the end of the week they get me onto my first red run, as thrilling and exhilarating an experience as I have ever had. We eat wonderfully, we sauna and soak, we play cards in the bar and endless games of Star Wars over dinner (you have to name characters, ships, vehicles or planets until you run out, whereupon you are out – a game can take several hours).

On the last day we go to the swimming pool in Canazei, a mighty and elegant complex where you can swim outside in steaming warm water under the gaze of the frozen mountains.

'Well,' Robin says and grins, delivering his verdict. 'A successful holiday. Who'd have thought it?'

We laugh joyfully. Everything Rebecca had hoped for us the first time has come true now, a year later. I thought about ending this book here, in the swimming pool under the snow, the sky dimming, the stars coming out, and all four of us deeply happy. But that would not be the full story.

January in Hebden is hard, as January always is. I miss my father terribly. The book is a fight. Returning to Manchester to teach is terrifying. On two nights, unable to sleep for fretting, I take a loxapine pill, the antipsychotic I was prescribed in France. As the French doctor said, if you cannot sleep, take one. It works, knocking me out.

Carefully and unconfidently, I go back to lecturing and teaching. Sessions with Jane are vital at this time – she teaches me simple, physical methods of defraying and reducing panic and stress.

'What is the worst that can happen?' she asks, and makes me ask myself. 'Even if they sack you, even if the book is no good, you are very resourceful. You will survive.'

Simple words, but all I am capable of understanding at the moment. On a notepad, Jane sketches a tolerance window, in which you can function. Too much stress produces a threat response, pushing you out of the window: you cannot sleep, cognitive and memory functions in the frontal cortex are impaired and now you cannot think. She does a sketch like an infinity symbol.

'Here, in the left-hand bubble, is the past. That is where the depressed spend their time, thinking about what went wrong. Here in the right bubble is the future – this is where you find the neurotic. But here, this little crossover, this junction, this is the present. This is where we actually are. You need to spend more time here. How often do you sit still and just . . . do nothing?'

'Not counting smoking? Not counting looking at a view because I am trying to describe it? Never.'

'You should try it,' Jane says. 'Try just . . . sitting, and doing nothing.'

Little by little, I come through. *There is nothing inexplicable about it*, I keep thinking. *You are definitely seasonally affective. A lot of work and pressure have come at the same time. You are missing your father very much. Hold fast, keep doing it.*

I do. The students are terrific. I can still teach. All will be well. I find that despite never having had open dialogue therapy, the ideas to which Yasmin Ishaq introduced me are powerfully effective in my everyday dealings with my students

and my family. My third-years at the university and my MA
students have all the usual worries of these pressured periods,
exacerbated this term by first the threat then the effect of
strikes, and the approaching menace of a new virus which
has emerged in China. I find myself trying out dialogical
approaches to teaching. Instead of trying to impersonate an
authority figure with answers to their stresses and uncertainties, I think about what Yasmin told me. I find myself saying,
'That is an absolutely understandable reaction to what you
are going through.' I aim to normalise their fears and uncertainties. In seminars I attempt to position us all in what
Yasmin called a flattened hierarchy: I try to create an environment in which all our voices have equal weight, an atmosphere of common endeavour in which we move forward as a
group, as one. I resist the temptation to defuse my own worries
by attempting to offer solutions. Instead, I make suggestions,
being candid about my worries and fears as the strikes, and
behind them the virus, close in. It works beautifully.

One winter night, coming back from the university on my
regular Monday commute through Manchester Victoria, I
stop at the bar which used to be the station restaurant. A
beautiful, arched exterior in glazed brick now contains a
nondescript pub. Inside, men and women are staring up at
a television screen showing the news. Figures in white
chemical-warfare suits are sealing the front door of a house.
'In the Chinese city of Wuhan,' the reporter's voice says,
'people infected with coronavirus are being isolated and quar-
antined indoors . . .'

We do not have television at home, though we take in a
great deal of news from the Internet and the radio.

'No wonder everyone is so worried,' I tell Rebecca that
night as we make supper. 'The pictures from China are
terrifying. It looks like the end of the world.'

Throughout January and February, I make regular visits
back to the ward in Wakefield, where I offer creative writing

sessions to the patients. It is not easy: levels of literacy diverge wildly, drugs and stress make it hard for the men to speak, and a member of staff must be present at all times. Susan, a support worker, is wonderfully unfettered and sympathetic, but her presence makes the men uncomfortable about talking freely. Little by little we work out how the sessions can be most effective. The men begin writing poems in their own time but in our sessions, they say, they just want to talk. They have no access to talking therapies.

'I am having CBT,' says one, 'but it's all about strategies for the future. What I want to do is talk about the past. About the good things and the bad, about what happened to put me in here.'

We use poems – Larkin, Hughes, Plath, Betjeman, D. H. Lawrence, Auden – as ways of starting conversations. We talk about good days and bad days. I write down what the men say and make simple poems out of their words in order to encourage them to do the same. Soon our regular group is just four: me, Matt, David and Susan. We sit outside when we can, in the first bright sun of the year, and try to talk as though there are no locks and no dread between us and the outside world.

I understand, now, why so many people who have suffered breakdowns become involved in the treatment of the unwell. Partly, being with people who are in crisis or recovering from crisis is reassuring: it tells me I must be sane, or at least more sane than they are, because I can leave whenever I want, because even when I am feeling shaky I am not as 'bad' as they are. And of course, my experiences do make it much easier for me to talk with the men, and therefore able to do some little good.

There is another reason too. I was formed as a child on a mountain sheep farm with my mother and brother, as teenager at college in Wales, as a student at university in York, as a young man by the BBC in London. But the person

I am and will be was partly made and remade in Wakefield. Even years hence, this ward will be part of me. Some part of me will never quite leave it, will never quite want to leave it, perhaps.

And I was lucky. I have interviewed people who underwent terrible abuse in locked wards in other cities. Our system has dreadful flaws, but although I have seen them and heard of them I have not been subject to them. If someone I loved had a psychotic breakdown tomorrow I would not hesitate to make the call which would lead to their sectioning, but I would keep a very close eye on their experiences, and, however mad, I would listen to what they told me about their ward and be ready to take any complaint they might make urgently to the highest level.

The last hands I shake before the news from China becomes the end of the world we knew are Matt's and David's in the hospital in Wakefield. Everyone is frightened now. The virus is on its way. Matt is being sent home, in stages, and he is scared he will not be able to cope. We try to reassure him. David will be discharged a week or so later. I am surprised. Neither seems ready for the world. They are heavily medicated and both say they struggle to leave their rooms. No doubt their clinicians have decided they stand a good chance of managing, and no doubt their beds are needed by men who are more unwell. We complete a joint poem; I merely arranged their words.

Everyman's Day on the Ward

Rattle of keys
Half seven cup of tea and a cig
A rollie. Right there by the no-smoking sign
And birds moving in the hedges.
Watch them. Look up.
Perfect sky.

Breakfast TV
Piers Morgan taking piss
Susanna Reid and banter
David's smiling.

8.45 Gary shouts *Breakfast*
Gary – his *voice*!
Matt's smiling.

Fry up and winding up the staff:
Alison and Charlotte need the joy.

When you get a massage
The touch
The warmth
The calm . . .

Meds?
To be the first in the queue is a good day.

You have to push yourself out of your room, sometimes
David says.
Matt nods.
We all feel it.
Push yourself out of the room.

As we talk in this last session, I try to reassure Matt that he will be OK, that there will be support, that the system is there to help him. He is terribly torn, desperate to see his daughter again and very fearful that he will not be able to cope. David shares his fear. David really only feels safe in his room. As we sit around a table in the small yard I understand and share the feeling of safety, of containment, that the ward provides. For all that I longed to be out of there when I was a patient, I realise now that it was and is a tiny, knowable world of fixed routines and little pressure except for whatever comes from within. As I speak, as I offer reassurances, I do not know if what I am saying is true. Is there really support available? Will it help? Can either of these men possibly expect to make a recovery on drugs they will take in ever greater quantities, which have been shown to mask symptoms but do nothing for their causes? Will they get the psychotherapy they both so obviously need and say they want?

I doubt it.

CHAPTER 36

The new world

We are standing on the roof of the moors, gazing at the horizon. It is some time in the afternoon, and it is May, but the date is uncertain, irrelevant. In a few dizzying days in March the entire world changed, and now I have the strange sense that the past and the future are folded into the present.

The light seems to belong to my childhood, sky-light, clean and fresh and clear for miles and miles. We can make out the details of trees and wind turbines in the far distance. There are curlews in the rough fields behind us. Below in the valley a cuckoo is calling. There are swallows diving and twittering around the high farms. The swifts are back. I watch them keenly in the evenings, before the bats come out.

Our lockdown routine is lovely. We work in the mornings, our boy enrolled in Rebecca's online school. I am busy with multiple commissions for pieces about nature and (in memory and imagination) travel. We are fit. Rebecca determines our regular walking route: through the meadow, through the woods, along the valley, over the stream, up on to the ridge and back on a wide ragged circle along the dreamy road which runs along the edge of the sky between the woods and the hilltop. Our son likes to stop at a certain tree, which he climbs. We eat apples and talk of many things. Later we will return to the house in time for the evening news on the radio.

We will pour wine and make supper. I will read our boy to sleep from *The Prisoner of Zenda* or *Peter Pan*.

I think of Dad a lot. I miss my brother and our mother. Mum seems to be enjoying what everyone calls the apocalypse. She has been predicting something like it for years; she relishes the absence of aeroplanes and traffic, the respite for the earth and the environment. And I miss my friends and travel, but really part of me wishes this utterly different life, with its peaceful beauty and the sense of all its present moments, would last and last for ever.

I am not lying any more. Early in lockdown an argument with Rebecca turned into a frank exchange. I admitted I was not taking the pills, had never really taken them, and said that I never would. Rebecca was hurt and infuriated by the deceit, but she accepted the obvious: I am well and have been well for a long time.

'If you don't take them for two or three years, and nothing happens, then . . .' Dr Y said when I asked him about rather than accepting the bipolar diagnosis and taking lithium, I should simply avoid cannabis, excess stress and sleeplessness.

One down, two to go.

The Covid crisis has brought a lurching rise in fear, depression, isolation and mental health pressures of all kinds. Yet at the same time it has broadened and deepened the national conversation about how we should best address these trials. Ideas that we are all on a continuum of mental well-being, that we all suffer without nature, rest, connection, the arts and mindful time in the outdoors – that we all have mental health and well-being needs – seem suddenly ubiquitous and obvious.

With the past strangely remote and the future unclear, the present is with us in astonishing fullness. Friends who suffer from anxiety and depression report that the quietening and slowing of the world has been a great balm to them. Some of the ways in which we used to live seem lunatic, unsustainable, harmful to ourselves and everything else. The protest that so many of the troubled, the young and the marginal make – that it is not us, but the world which is mad – has rarely seemed to make so much sense.

In writing this book, there were moments when I could not bear to look too long at things I did. The hells I and Rebecca and our children went through I will carry with me. And although this is a hopeful story of progress into healing, I can make no claim that my shadows are banished; it will not necessarily be all right in the end. I shall have to wait and see.

Although what happened and what I did often brought out the worst in me, time and again my chaos and destruction brought out the best in others, and so I end this account with the most profound and humble sense of gratitude and admiration for my family, my friends, my town and all who dealt with me and spoke to me.

At times, researching and recounting this, I have felt fury on behalf of those in distress for the way our system treats them. It is not for me to tell anyone how they should address their suffering, but my most solemn advice would be to beware of the kind of psychiatry I encountered. Comparing how I am now with how I would have been with a year of aripiprazole inside me, and how I might have been with years of lithium ahead of me, makes me feel as though I dodged a hail of chemical bullets.

It was wrong that I was not listened to, and it was wrong that my request for a second opinion met only incredulity. It was wrong that I should have had to rely on luck and persistence to find a psychiatrist, Peter Macrae, who was prepared to listen to what I was saying and to admit the possibility of another narrative. And it is most grievously wrong that the treatments which made all the difference to me, psychotherapy and EMDR, should not be available free and quickly to any who might benefit from them, a great many of whom cannot afford sixty pounds an hour.

Were I taking pills now, I would press for an appointment with my GP and ask insistently about strategies for coming off them safely. Regular therapy would have to be a central part of those strategies. I would recognise that our under-standing and treatment of mental disorders are still in their infancies. I would tell myself not to be frightened by the language or by the reams of doom available on the Internet. Put psychiatry under a little pressure, and much of it turns out to be guesswork, formulaic thinking, generalisation and trial and error. You are what you are, and there is no pill for that. There is no pill for the causes of your symptoms.

I have little patience with the *Diagnostic and Statistical Manual*'s understanding of the unique circumstances and pressures suffered by the millions of people who are prescribed pills on the strength of its edicts. Until the wording changed in its fourth edition in 1980, I would have been diagnosed with manic depression. Now the dread phrase is bipolar disorder. I find it so general as to be useless.

Bipolar, we are told, runs in families. My father suffered depressions. There was nothing inexplicable about them: he endured abuse from his mother, estrangement from his father, a long series of failed relationships, perfectionism, work pres-sure and great loneliness. My sister (technically my half-sister, my father's first child) committed suicide. Janey was trauma-tised by Dad's divorce from her mother, by his absence thereafter, by heavy drug use in her teens and twenties, by unemployment in later life, by poverty and by isolation, all of which led to terrible feelings of guilt and marginalisation. And though no gene has been identified for bipolar, my psychiatrists saw a big ticked box when I said one family member had been depressed and another had killed herself. As Yasmin Ishaq put it, my psychiatrists' curiosity as to what might actually be wrong with me was further reduced: the *DSM* in action again.

The kind of psychotherapy, trauma counselling and EMDR which so helped me would have changed my father's and my sister's lives, unquestionably. My story shows that I underwent a series of highs and lows, culminating in a breakdown, which all had the same causes: life events, habitual and dangerous ways of thinking and acting, and disastrous levels of alcohol and especially cannabis use, to which I am notably vulnerable. Identify the harmful thought patterns, address the underlying trauma, remove the cannabis, establish positive strategies of behaviour (sleep, exercise, diary management, honesty in relationships) and what do you get?

You get me. You get someone who feels and appears to be a normal and fortunate man. There have been miracles here aplenty, in kindness and luck and love and support, but there was no mystery.

We count our blessings. Rebecca, our son and Robin and I go to sleep peacefully and wake up hopeful, with plans. Regrettably but necessarily, I am planning to go a little mad again. I promised our boy that when this book is finished I will give up smoking. I will be a rapid-cycling, depressed, volatile nightmare for the first three weeks, but after that things will get better. Fortunately, we still have the flat, so I will partly quarantine myself there while I go through it.

Over a year since Chris cleaned them, the windows need doing again. Beyond them, the sky has never been so bright, the horizon so sharp, the air so clear and lucent. While the summer lasts I will watch the swifts slicing and screaming over the roofs of Hebden at twilight. Some nights, when I cannot sleep, the barn owl will fly past. I saw her the other evening and she turned her head towards me. My breath caught. Imagine perceiving as she does! A hundred times more sensitive to light than we are, she registers fewer colours. But her world is an unfurling spectrum of nuanced greys and textures of black. Perhaps, seeing me staring out of the window, she registered an ordinary man, earth-bound, no threat, doing nothing.

Acknowledgements

This story is a poor thanks for great kindnesses. Loath, usually, to strain a reader's patience, I make no apology for these notes, though they are inadequate.

Zoë Waldie, my agent at Rogers, Coleridge and White, guided and helped to shape this book, flawlessly assisted by Miriam Tobin. Thank you, dear Miriam. Thank you, dear Zoë, for so much over the years. You really are the best: wise counsellor, wonderful friend, simply brilliant agent.

Becky Hardie, my editor at Chatto & Windus, faced with a man in a rocky place with difficult material, was unwavering in her belief, her judgement and her understanding. Given a half-chaotic mess of a manuscript, she produced the kind of edit and the kind of guidance for which any writer would pray. I cannot thank you enough, dear Becky.

Any infelicities, errors and deficiencies contained herein are entirely mine, and in no way reflect the tremendous skill and professionalism of all those at Chatto who worked on this book. To the peerless woman behind it all, Publishing Director Clara Farmer, to copy-editor Hugh Davis and assistant editor Greg Clowes, to designer Matt Broughton (who created the knock-out cover) to tireless and terrific publicist Christian Lewis – *thank you*. It is an honour to be your writer.

Sincere thanks to Anne Farthing, Peter Macrae, Marge Mather, Ellen Sieg, Yasmin Ishaq, Brigid Bowen, Matt

Walsh, Robin Tuddenham, Salma Yasmeen, Christine Brown, Dickie Whitehead, Carol Harris, Zoe Akesson, Ben Owens, Tim Mellard and the staff of the ward for your help, your expertise, your time and trouble.

Thank you, John McAuliffe, sublime leader and friend; thank you, tirelessly kind Kaye Mitchell and thank you, all my friends at the Centre for New Writing at the University of Manchester – especially Honor Gavin and Ian McGuire, who did extra hours – for your support and understanding of a colleague breaking down. From our wonderful heads of department – then Peter Knight and now Hal Gladfelder – to John and Kaye and Jeanette Winterson, to my students and my partner in crime (non-fiction section) Cathy Miller, the way you handled and helped me throughout the crisis and its aftermaths was exemplary, and humbling. Thank you.

In Wales, thank you Roger Couhig, Nic Shugar, Niall Griffiths and Deborah Jones, for your complete friendship, your easy understanding, your magnificent example and your ever-open doors. Try as I might, you are impossible to phase, surprise or alarm. Thank you.

In Liverpool, thank you Jeff Young! Extraordinary friend, mentor, hero, spell-caster, the Kafka of Merseyside – cheers mate.

In Rochdale, thank you, as ever, Jennifer Shooter. You put up with horrors from me with utter steadiness and kindness. You look after all of us, all of the time. I apologise from the bottom of my heart for being such a hideous monster and causing you (and so many named here) such pain and worry. Thank you Gerald Shooter, Emma Shooter, Matthew and Jennifer Divine, Scott Tetlow, Gail Tetlow, Kate Burns, Bernard Burns and Sandra and David Wright. You do what Rochdalians seem to do so naturally and so magnificently: standing together and supporting (and carrying, when necessary) friends and family – with such steadfastness, love and respect. I have not always been worthy to stand in your company but I am deeply honoured and grateful to be part of your – our – amazing family. No thanks could be anywhere near adequate – but, thank you. It was particularly awful to be in your position, Scott, with your son Robin so confronted with and distressed by my madness – and for all you knew, endangered by it. Typically, you were absolutely kind and wise, and forgiving. Thank you, sir.

Chris Shooter was a complete rock when I was sectioned, sending extraordinary kindness in your messages. Thank you, dear Chris.

Thank you Bushra Sultana, Alistair Bennett, Caroline Flinders, Stuart and Jade, Miriea Griffiths, Jud and Esther Greenwood, Jody Trick and Kremena Krasteva, Jeremy Grange, Kevin Bohnert, Robin Jenkins, Graham Da Gama Howells and the BBC Zoom boys, Alison 'Tig' Finch, friends near and far and ever incredibly kind.

I am deeply fortunate in the friendship of extraordinary companions in the world of writing. Messages, calls, travels or conversations with Merlin and Anna Rose Hughes, Douglas Field, Jonty Driver, Jay Griffiths, Robert Macfarlane, Kapka Kassabova, Jon Gower, Anna Gavalda, Dan Richards, Niall Griffiths, Julia Bell, Kaye Mitchell, Zaffar Kunial, Ben Myers, Laura Barton, John McAuliffe, Sian and Ceri Phillips, Peter Florence, Becky Shaw, Sophy Roberts and Jeff Young are the true treasure of this job: lifelines in crisis, lights in any darkness, singers of the great song, thank you. (And golly you do make it *fun* . . .)

In Hebden Bridge, thank you Doug Field, Ellie Field, Zaffar Kunial, Phil O'Farrell, Emma Back, Vicky Bloomfield, Jayn Macnamara, Benjamin Myers, Fiona Windsor, Jack Bell, Jill Penny, the famous and astonishing Peter and Leah Findlay, and all on our road Gary and Suzanne, Martine and Pete, Jan and Femi, Lyndon, Bernadette, Liz, Sonya and Giles. Your kindness embodies the very special spirit of our town. Thank you.

Emma Back came out in the middle of the night to help a lunatic in a police station. Doug and Ellie gave awe-inspiring support and help to Rebecca and me and our family. You are the very souls of friendship. Thank you.

Thank you particularly, dearest Doug, for the socks, the crocs, the advice, the humour, the gifts, for sorting my sicknote, for the visit with Ellie, for holding so many forts for all of us, for *everything* you do and did for the boys and for us.

Dear amazing Ellie Field, thank you!

Chris Kenyon, Richard Coles and Diarmaid Gallagher dropped everything and came to the rescue. Thank you, you extraordinary men. May you reap all you so generously sow, so lightly, so reliably, with such love and care and wicked humour. You will find each other hard to avoid in Heaven. Chris will be the one organising it; Diarmaid will be making the jokes; Richard will be the angels' confessor.

My family, Sally Clare, Alexander Clare, Roy and Sarah Clare, Cynthia Clare, Anthea Robinson, Robin Tetlow-Shooter, Rebecca Shooter and The Bug cannot be properly thanked in words. Thank you, Roy and Sarah, and thank you, dear Cindy. Your support is wonderful, always. And thank you, dear Anthea.

Robin Christopher Tetlow-Shooter: you are extraordinary, dear Robin. I cannot say how much I admire your grace or how much I appreciate your forbearance and your kindness.

Thank you, dearest Ma. (How can one even begin, dear mother?)

Thank you, dearest A. What a mighty loving brother you are.

Rebecca Shooter; there are still no words. Thank you, my love.

And because you were always there, and will always be here, thank you, John Clare, dearest Dad. Here's another one for your shelf. (The next will be more fun, I promise.)

With all my love – H x x